HEART ATTACK
SURVIVOR

D1562374

Here's what readers are saying about
Heart Attack Survivor – a field guide:

As a financial advisor for many years, I can see the benefits of keeping your debt under control and having it not control you, which Brad brings forth in his book Heart Attack Survivor – a field guide. This is sound financial advice that I would give any of my clients."

Scott R. Alexander, MBA, Registered Financial Advisor, Chartered Financial Consultant, and Chartered Life Underwriter.

"I have read this book cover to cover and found it to be VERY uplifting to both mind and spirit. I only wish there had been a book like this when my Dad had his heart attack. Thanks Brad, for taking the time to help all of us, not just the Heart Attack survivors. I came away a better person."

Candy Finn, Ventura, California

"Heart Attack Survivor - a field guide" is a wonderful book, full of wisdom. The author helps the reader to slow down the inner engine, so as to make it possible to feel and live life in a way for which we were called. This book is heartwarming, filled with real life stories, told with humor, love, and insight. Heart Attack Survivor should be on everyone's night-stand.

**Stephan Ogenstad, Ph.D.
Professor of Statistics**

"Brad tells his story with passion and personality. This book is filled with practical ideas, humor and inspiration. It will be a useful tool for anyone who needs to de-stress."

**Nancy Paul, M.A., Marriage & Family Therapist
Ventura, California**

HEART ATTACK
SURVIVOR
a field guide

So you survived...NOW what??

BRAD HENSON, MBA/TM

Crow Publishing
Camarillo, California

Printed in the United States of America.

For information address:
Crow Publishing
2510-G Las Posas Rd. #260
Camarillo, California 93010
www.heartattacksurvivor.com
bhenson@heartattacksurvivor.com

Library of Congress Control Number: 2001119212

Henson, Brad, 1950 April 7 -
Heart Attack Survivor- a field guide
So you survived - NOW what? / Brad Henson
p. cm.

1. Health   2. Success   3. Business people-Conduct of life
4. Happiness   5. Self-actualization (Psychology)
6. Job satisfaction   7. Work-Psychological aspects.

Paperback ISBN: 0-9712788-0-6

FIRST PAPERBACK EDITION
1 3 5 7 9 10 8 6 4 2

Book design by Bookcovers.com

DEDICATION

THIS BOOK IS DEDICATED TO BETH, MY WIFE,
BEST FRIEND, CONFIDANTE, LOVER, AND ADVISOR
WITHOUT WHOM NEITHER THIS BOOK...
SURVIVAL, AND EVENTUAL NO-LIMIT LIFESTYLE
WOULD HAVE BEEN POSSIBLE.

THANK YOU FOR YOUR EVERLASTING LOVE,
GENEROSITY, GUIDANCE AND CREATIVE IDEAS

I LOVE YOU

♥   ♥   ♥

This book is also dedicated to the other true survivors of heart disease - the men and women who are the significant others of the survivors, the husbands, wives, girl and boy friends and children of YOU, the person who had the heart attack. These people are the witnesses to the single most devastating event in their loved one's lives, and these people are the ones who have stood by, encouraged, supported, and loved you while you were recovering from your stay in the hospital. This is my way of saying "Thank You" for your love and devotion while I, and now you, rise like a Phoenix to live that NO-Limit life you have always deserved.

I don't need to know everything

♥   ♥   ♥

Just what's important

CONTENTS

FOREWORD

Everyone who has survived a heart attack has many questions about what can be done to regain a strong sense of health, and have a vibrant life. But who is there every day to give you real answers? After a heart attack, your whole life changes forever. You realize that you now have new mental physical and emotional challenges to conquer. At times, you feel as though you are scaling a high wall of apprehension and fear. Some days, you'll battle mountainous anger as you ask yourself why a heart attack had to happen to you. You'll experience confusion as your mind races to sort out conflicting information about what to do to reduce your risk of a future heart attack. This book is about conquering the self-inflicted "mind games" that will try to ensnare you and finding fast actionable answers to your most pressing questions. Here you will find sensible solutions for making changes that will help you live a balanced, happy and long life.

Brad Henson wrote this book to remind you that you're not alone. Brad successfully survived a heart attack at age 35. He had been a corporate guerilla fighter, battling lethal opposition in his own self-induced version of a corporate war. Brad unknowingly allowed stress, over-work, and mental as well as emotional life imbalance to take their toll on him. The day Brad had a heart attack was the day he became a casualty in the very corporate war in which he fought hard to gain recognition. On that day, Brad lay alone in an emergency room as he was brought back to life with not one of his fellow corporate soldiers by his side. From that day forward, Brad began learning how to make what he later called simple "Heart Attack Survivor Life-Changes" the result of a two-decade search for real-life answers. This book is the fruit of Brad's hunt to rebuild a better, more fulfilling life than before his heart attack. Heart Attack Survivor - a field guide gives you solid answers to practical questions based on an every day approach to medical, psychological, nutritional, and other profound multi-discipline-based principles. Now in his 50s, Brad enjoys a fun, enriching, purposeful, energetic, and confident life - a life he has created using the fundamentals he has distilled in the contents of this book.

If your heart attack occurred recently, Heart Attack Survivor -a field guide, will become your constant companion. As you read this book, you will learn new things about yourself, personality type, and life patterns that you have unknowingly developed, which increase your risk of a heart attack. You will realize that now is the time to consider making some wonderfully radical changes in thought and action to save your life and make it better. It is time to learn from those who have been where you are now and have successfully conquered to move from "heart attack survivors" to "whole life thrivers."

Allen D'Angelo,
Archer-Ellison, January 2002

ACKNOWLEDGEMENTS

I want to express my love to my family for their never-ending support, understanding, and patience during my journey of writing this book.

To my Children - Bill Walling, Jr., Kelly Imber, Kimberly Sanabria, and Noelle Henson, and Grandchildren - Anthony, Jr., Abby Beth, Bridgette, Denna, Joshua, Kathy, Kyle, Jade, and Jessica: For continually reminding me you are *never* to old to learn, play, and laugh, love and be loved.

To my parents - Robert and Corinne Patrick – "Thank you" for providing me with the necessary tools needed to survive out in the "real world".

A special dedication to Will Gamble, whose love of all things great and small will never be forgotten by those who had the honor and privilege of knowing him. "Thank you" for your kindness, understanding, and always finding time to answer my questions.

A special dedication to both my grandmothers – Leona Henson, and Ottie Gamble, for just being yourselves. Thanks for your great stories and heartfelt and ageless guidance and wisdom, which now is an integrated part of who I am.

A special dedication to my Uncle, Jim Grier – who taught me to wonder at the world's magnificence, and who educated me in the fine art of "Cat fish'n".

I sincerely want to take this time to thank all the wonderful people that assisted in making this book possible. Thank you for your honesty, generosity, time, immense talent, and love for what is a very important endeavor.

Candy Finn – To my dear friend - for her boundless energy, hope springs eternal optimism, and honestly straight answers to very deep questions.

Nancy Paul – Marriage and Family Counselor – for the years of friendship, encouragement, advice and counsel.

Dr. Scott Alexander, The Alexander Group of Financial Planning - for being a mentor and master teacher at the beginning of my journey through the gauntlet called academia.

Mr. Richard Hatch, Actor – "Thank You" for teaching me to listen, and to trust my "inner voice" for the answers to my most difficult questions.

To my brother, Greg – for you are truly my greatest hero. Be at peace.

DISCLAIMERS

I have written, designed and published this book to give you information in regards to the subject matter, which I have covered between the front and back cover. I am selling this work with the clear understanding that neither I, nor the publisher, will be engaged in giving out legal, medical, or other professional services. If you desire any of the above-mentioned services, please obtain advice from competent professionals in your local area.

I have made every effort to make this book as accurate as possible and as complete as time allows. However, unfortunately, there may be mistakes...both in content and/or typography, and because of this eventuality, the book should only be utilized as a general source of knowledge and not the ultimate resource to universal knowledge on these subjects for which I have written. Please note that the book contains data only up to the printed date.

The journey for answers...upon which you have embarked, is a fun, fulfilling, and joyous adventure, and this book only gives one man's opinion on how to better reach some sound conclusions, which you seek. Remember, it's not a get-well-quick scheme. Anyone who reads this book must expect to invest many thought-provoking hours to this new path...hopefully to come out the other side a changed and better person because of it.

If you don't want to be bound by the above, you may return this book to the publisher for a FULL refund.

INTRODUCTION

Heart Disease. Just the very mention of the words conjure up feelings of despair, anxiety, and fear. As we move into the 21st century, the world is becoming more complex in its makeup, and the inhabitants are growing further and further apart, physically, emotionally, as well as spiritually...and there is no end in sight. We are fleeing the cities for the suburbs, and leaving our homelands to live halfway around the world. We think the Internet, phone and fax will keep our families close and the vast transportation networks are there whenever we feel a need to visit our friends, relatives, and co-workers. The days when the family unit was within close proximity to each other has long fallen away. A time when family members were close enough to help each other when another family member needed assistance has long disappeared.

That time in our history is gone, replaced with telephones, pagers, fax machines, cell phones, and video conferencing. All of these "tools", no matter how advanced and sophisticated they have become, can't take the place of a "hug", a kiss, or intimate conversations between family members while sitting on the porch of the family home on a hot summer's night, or at the kitchen table over a hot cup of coffee.

As we become more distant from our loved ones and scatter out in the great global village we now live in, more and more everyday stress of living creeps into our lives...partly due to us not having the proper tools, or techniques, at our fingertips, to defuse it. With corporate downsizing, rightsizing, mergers and acquisitions, divorce, and more and more people becoming members of fractured family units, these changes are occurring at a faster and faster pace as time goes by. Normalcy is being replaced with uncertainty and chaos, and no one has effectively taught us how to deal with these changes. This escalating level of stress has nowhere to go, and eventually manifests itself in increased levels of frustration and anger, slowly tearing down the body's immune system. The cascade effect(tm) of all this chaos shows up in higher and higher rates of obesity, cancer, high blood pressure, and stress-related heart disease.

Over the years since my stress-induced heart attack, and ultimate rebirth, I developed an insatiable appetite for learning the root cause of me ending up dead on a hospital gurney. My need to know was not just tied to the "how" of the heart attack, but more to the "why." I wanted to find out how I fit into this great big world of ours, and how I could stay in it for a much longer time.

It has been a journey of the spirit, laden with successes, and also with failures along the way. Through it all, and coming out the other end, I feel I am far better off today than when I started, with the knowledge I have acquired.

This book is written to show how to establish new behavior patterns. I am writing this as a field guide, like a Boy Scout or Girl Scout would take with him or her on an outing into the woods. Remembering my Boy Scout adventures as a youth reminds me of all those weekends away at "camp". As a mandatory piece of equipment, along with a metal, water-resistant match holder, a flashlight, and compass, we carried our trusted Boy Scout Field Guide. In that trusted piece of gear was every answer to almost all eventualities that might occur when out in the "rough", facing dangers from unseen threats to our safety.

I hope you look at, and treat this, with the same reverence as I did my Field Guide all those years ago, by referring to it whenever you get in trouble or want to refresh yourself with the answers to your questions about how not to have another episode like you've had.

My attempt with this book is to show you ways to re-establish balance in your life, and remove any and all poisonous toxins from the heart muscle and replace it with the "elixir of life."

My hope is that this book and commentary will do a number of things for you, as it has for me, by putting my trials and tribulations down on paper. I have had to openly admit that I had fears and doubts about things that happened to me. I then had to examine them from all angles. I have seen the cause of my heart problem, and the cause was "me." During my research, I was taken to areas of the human mind I didn't know existed until my journey began, some fifteen years ago. Through it all, I have started to piece together a "roadmap" that...up to now, did not exist.

My desire for you, my friends...is to digest parts of, if not all, of this information with an open mind, heart and soul, taking away the knowledge you are looking for. My hope is that you will share your fears, desires, and dreams with your loved ones, as a way for them to see into your life after you emerged victoriously from your disease. Perhaps they will understand things about your strange behavior, silence, and mood swings (like I exhibited), and then engage them in a partnership with you, toward a full and triumphant recovery. If it was not for my wife,

Beth, and her love and wisdom for me in my time of pain, I do not believe I would be here today to pass on this information.

What this book is not

I have kept this book as light and as airy as possible in its view and conversation about Heart Disease. I am sure that by now, you have listened to your doctors, nurses, and/or Cardiologists about what caused the problem that changed your life until you are blue in the face, and would love to go on with your life.

The sole purpose of this book is to provide encouragement for you to get out of your own way and live a wonderful, enlightened life. As the title states, "So you survived - Now what?"

This book is not a dictionary of medical terms, or information about the prevention of heart disease. There are tons of books on that subject already on the market, and this is not one of them. This book is full of life-changing concepts and fresh new ideas, as well as humorous anecdotes, and as many inspirational stories as I could cram into this limited dissertation from people that have become survivors and thrived after a life-threatening disease. I have also included fun things to get you to start thinking about how valuable life really is. Think of this as a "Readers Digest" for the heart!!! A practical life management skills field guide full of solutions to the common (and not so common) issues surrounding heart disease.

Enjoy the information, but don't take it too seriously. That's what got me into trouble in the first place. Put it on the nightstand and read it at your leisure, digesting little bits of its contents every day until it has been read completely. Give it to the other members of your family to read and get feedback from them on its contents. Start a dialogue with the ones that matter the most to you about what really happened to you. I have provided my email and address so you can send me comments about the contents, so I, too, can learn, because we are all in this together.

I have provided both a 50,000 foot view and an "in the trenches Field Guide" to the subject of surviving and THRIVING after heart disease. At the end of each chapter are anecdotes and stories that have been gathered over the years from people all over the world. Most of them came from family members who received them from other people who received them from other people. Most, if not all, are anonymous authors, so credit is not possible on an individual basis. I want to take this opportunity now to "Thank" each and every one of you...whoever and wherever you are.

- Brad Henson -

"Live long and prosper"
- Mr. Spock- USS Enterprise
From the TV series - Star Trek

CHAPTER 1

The Story- A second chance at life

I have two birthdays. The first was April 7, 1950. My second was August 16, 1985. That's the day I had my heart attack. I was 35 years of age at the time.

It was your classic heart attack. I was having dinner with my wife and a friend at a local restaurant when the pain started in my left fingers and spread up my arm into my chest, tightening like a vise. On the way to the hospital, I basically died in the back of the car...being clinically dead until they revived me with those electric paddles. People always ask how long I was gone. The only answer is "long enough."

When I regained consciousness, a cardiologist was standing over me with a clipboard. He started running down a checklist of lifestyle factors that cause heart attacks. The first question was "How much alcohol do you drink?" I told him I didn't drink at all. Then "How much do you smoke?" I don't smoke. "What about drugs?" I don't do drugs and never have. Period.

The doctor looked up from his clipboard, with a puzzled look on his face. I was not making this easy. I wanted to understand why he was asking these questions of a 35-year-old man who didn't drink, smoke, or do drugs, and who had no history of heart problems. He was baffled. Finally he just said "Then, why the hell are you here?"

Good question. What did cause my heart attack?

In a word, "stress". In 1985, I was employed, and trying to move up the corporate ladder. Unfortunately, I was selling IBM typewriters in a world that was moving into computers. The fact that I was carrying around 240 pounds of weight on my body frame that should have been only carrying 195 pounds didn't help either. I knew I was about 45 pounds overweight, ...but I had always been a little on the heavy side. Besides, I was very active. Before my heart attack, I was actually running long distances on a daily basis, so I thought I was in really great shape.

There's nothing like death to give you a new perspective on life. You get a lot of time to think while you watch your vital signs on the monitors next to your hospital bed. The way I saw it, I was getting a second chance at life. I had to lose the stress, change my life, or not do anything, accept things as they were, and perhaps die a second time...for good. It was a matter of survival.

Lowering my stress was the easy part. I quit my job while I was still in the hospital. The moment I did, the monitor showed my blood pressure decreasing by 20 points.

As the old Chinese proverb states so eloquently "The journey of a thousand miles starts with the first step." My journey started with the first heartbeats being heard... once revived {and the beat goes on...}.

I have never seen a U-Haul attached to the rear of a hearse. In other words..."You can't take it with you... so don't even try."
        - Candy Finn -

CHAPTER 2

Why ME?
Tough problems are only given to those that can handle them

Sometimes I wonder..."why me?" What did I ever do to deserve heart disease? Over the years, I have had the chance to ask that question, over and over again. I have looked at it from every direction. From the point of an angry person, a scared person, a young man, a now older (than young) man, a husband, a father, son, corporate executive, grandfather, friend, and just a guy who had a life-changing event, and then ultimately from the point-of-view of one who has fully accepted the event in the overall universal plan for my life.

Someone told me once that we are given "no more than we can handle."

Throughout history, men and women have been asking the question, "why me?", when dealt a hand that they did not expect to be dealt. I can imagine the conversation that Noah must have had with God on that all too famous day in biblical history when God asked this simple man to build an Ark. Standing next to his tool shed, Noah looked up and stated emphatically - "Why me? WHY ME? I am just a simple man of simple means." I can just hear God's calm and reassuring voice replying, "Noah, I have chosen you for this all important job - because I KNOW you can make it happen. You have it within you to build this ARK."

In the quiet moments that Abe Lincoln must have experienced, sitting in the White House while contemplating his now famous speech before addressing the nation on his decision to abolish slavery, most likely turned to his wife and trusted advisor, and asked "Why me? Why have I been given the task of carrying the entire weight of this new nation on my shoulders? There has to be others than can do this job better than I." Can you hear his wife saying quietly and firmly "Abe, It IS self evident all men are not created equally - and that you have been given a task that only you can handle."

History demonstrates wonderful and inspirational stories of ordinary people who rise to the occasion and do extraordinary things when life tosses them a curve ball, and their lives don't turn out the way they thought it should. Perhaps the answer is that we are not given ONLY what we can handle. People like Noah, Abe, you, and me were given the bigger problems, because I believe that tough problems are given only to the best problem solvers.

If you believe that the universe has a "plan" for our lives, maybe we should look at it in a positive way - that we were handed a bad hand of cards, but, in a "good hand" not yet realized.

If I hadn't had the heart attack, I would not be the person I am today. I have become more aware of my strengths and limitations. I am convinced that if I had continued on the path I was on...when I had my heart attack, I would not be the strong, vital person I am today. I would be an out-of-control, angry, depressed, and hateful individual. The fact be known, if I had not stepped up to the challenge that was given to me, I probably would be dead today.

I made the decision, and I am a much happier person today.

As I continued on the new path of discovery I dug deep into my soul, fully accepted what had happened to me, and then started the most wonderful journey one could embark on - a path of self-discovery and change. Like a caterpillar morphing into a butterfly, I changed, and became better than I was before. I looked at this event as an opportunity to better myself, and change the direction of my destiny. It was a wake-up call for me and perhaps can be for you, as well. Opportunities (both good and bad) can be seen as either dead end streets, or as trials to be handled, gotten through and triumphed over.

If we accept the same attitude that the great leaders like Noah and Abraham Lincoln did, we, too, can rise to the occasion and accept what happened to us, and conquer this disease with gusto.

Just think about it!!!

♥   ♥   ♥

Contributed by Candy Finn, 2001
In honor of her dad

I WAS A MILITARY BRAT GROWING UP. MY FATHER WAS A CAREER AIR FORCE CHIEF MASTER SERGEANT AND WE HAD LIVED ALL OVER THE WORLD THROUGH MANY OF THE WORLD'S CHANGES. MY DAD WAS AN ACTIVE SOLDIER IN WORLD WAR II AND THE KOREAN CONFLICT. HE WAS NOT AFRAID OF ANYTHING. ONCE WE KIDS WERE PART OF THE SCENE, WE LIVED THROUGH THE CUBAN MISSILE CRISIS, THE ASSASSINATION OF PRESIDENT KENNEDY, THE IRANIAN HOSTAGE CRISIS, AND MANY OTHER FEARFUL THREATS AGAINST THE UNITED STATES AND ITS CITIZENS. TO MY SIBLINGS AND MYSELF, OUR DAD WAS INVINCIBLE.

IN THE LATE 1960'S, WE WERE LIVING IN GERMANY AND, ONCE AGAIN, MY DAD RECEIVED ORDERS THAT SIM-

PLY FLOORED US. I WAS ONLY 16 YEARS OLD AND MY DAD WAS BEING SENT TO THE FRONT IN VIETNAM! NEEDLESS TO SAY, WE WERE ALL SHOCKED, NERVOUS, SAD AND SCARED. DAD, AS USUAL, TOOK IT IN STRIDE AND PREPARED TO DO WHAT HE HAD TO DO TO DEFEND OUR COUNTRY. I PRAYED AND PRAYED TO GOD TO FIND A WAY TO LET DAD OFF THE HOOK. I SELFISHLY ASKED FOR HIM TO SEND OTHERS IN DAD'S PLACE, OR TO LOSE HIS ORDERS, OR TO JUST MAKE THE WAR GO AWAY. YOU CAN IMAGINE HOW SHOCKED I WAS WHEN I WAS SITTING IN 6TH PERIOD HISTORY, AT THE AMERICAN HIGH SCHOOL, AND SOMEONE FROM THE PRINCIPAL'S OFFICE CAME IN AND GAVE MY TEACHER A NOTE ASKING ME TO COME TO THE PRINCIPAL'S OFFICE RIGHT AWAY! I HAD NO IDEA WHAT WAS WRONG, BUT KNEW IN MY HEART THAT IT WASN'T GOOD NEWS. I AL-MOST RAN TO THE OFFICE.

WHEN I GOT THERE, MY MOTHER WAS STANDING THERE IN TEARS. SHE TOLD ME THAT MY FATHER HAD JUST HAD A MAJOR HEART ATTACK AND WAS RUSHED TO THE LOCAL MILITARY HOSPITAL. MY HEART SEEMED TO FALL TO THE FLOOR. I DIDN'T HAVE THE NERVE TO ASK IF HE WAS STILL ALIVE. I CAN'T TELL YOU HOW MANY VARIED THOUGHTS FLEW THROUGH MY MIND IN THE SECONDS THAT FOLLOWED. THE BEST NEWS WAS THE DAD WAS STILL ALIVE!

WE RUSHED OVER TO THE HOSPITAL WHERE MY DAD WAS IN INTENSIVE CARE. I WAS AFRAID OF WHAT I WOULD SEE WHEN WE ENTERED HIS ROOM. ALTHOUGH IT WAS SCARY SINCE HE WAS ATTACHED TO ALL KINDS OF TUBES AND MONITORS, WHEN MY DAD LOOKED AT ME AND MOUTHED "I LOVE YOU", I KNEW THE WORLD WAS GOING TO BE OKAY AGAIN. THE DOCTOR SAID HE WAS GOING TO BE FINE, BUT THAT HIS ORDERS TO VIETNAM WOULD HAVE TO BE CANCELLED DUE TO MEDICAL REASONS!

MY DAD RECOVERED AND LIVED ANOTHER FIFTEEN YEARS AFTER THAT FATEFUL HEART ATTACK. HE OFTEN

MENTIONED TO US THAT IT WAS THE LUCKIEST HEART AT-
TACK ANYONE COULD HAVE SINCE IT SPARED HIM FROM
ACTIVE DUTY ON THE FRONT IN VIETNAM. HE WAS CON-
VINCED THAT GOD, IN SOME WAY, HAD INTERVENED. EV-
ERY TIME I THINK BACK ON THOSE DAYS, I THANK GOD
FOR THE HEART ATTACK THAT SAVED MY DAD FROM LEAV-
ING US TO GO TO VIETNAM.

CHAPTER 3

Life is like a checkbook©
Live every day to the fullest

Years ago, when I was a bit younger than I am now, and just out of high school, I had dreams of working for the Federal Bureau of Investigation as a fingerprints expert. It sounded really "cool" to examine fingerprints left by the bad guys at crime scenes, capture them...and to protect the world from those that would do the world harm. I got interested in this because a police officer friend of mine pointed out that there are no two finger-prints that are the same...in the entire world. I didn't really realize the impact of that until years later, in 1985, when I had my heart attack. Lying in the hospital with lots of time on my hands allowed me to contemplate "life" and what had just happened to me. I remember clearly glancing down at my fingertips and remembering what that officer had said about being one-of-a-kind in this universe. At that moment, I realized that if I was the only person in the universe that had fingerprints that were so unique that no one else had ones like them, that I must be incredibly valuable, because of this unique-ness. The "insight" and flash of inspiration drove home the concept of placing a value on every single day that we are alive... and making that value the largest value possible.

Being in corporate life for the last 20 years or so, I have learned to see value...in the form of dollars spent or value gained. While I was lying on my back glancing up at the bare ceiling in the hospital's critical care unit, the concept of "Life is like a checkbook(c)" popped into my mind. It goes like this:

Yesterday is a cancelled check - it had a value, you can look and dream about how much the check was worth and the enjoyment that you derived from it. In reality, the check is now worthless. You can't use it for anything. It had worth. You can pull it out and touch it, feel it, smell it and dream about how much value and enjoyment the check gave you at the time, but it is now just a memory. Conversely, tomorrow is a promissory note. You can put a value on it. You can dream about how much it will be worth... but in reality, it, too, has no value...YET.

Today is a blank check. You can touch and feel it - right now. But more importantly, you can put a tangible value on it at this moment. My recommendation is that you place the largest value on the blank check today... and make it a HUGE one. The reality is we only have "this moment" and no others. There are absolutely no guarantees that anyone we will be around in the future. None.

The value you place on the check is equivalent to the worth and value you place on yourself. What are you worth? If you don't feel you are entitled to a huge dollar amount on that blank check... ask those around you - that really matter to you, what they think you are worth to them. Start with your family, friends, spouse, significant other, children, grandchildren and relatives. You may be blown away with what they have to say. I know that if I were to ask any one of my ten grandchildren that question, they would say there is not enough money in the "whole wide world" that could replace me.

We tend to take for granted how much we contribute to those around us on a day-to-day basis. I am not referring as much to the financial aspects of our lives, but more to the "content" of our lives in respect to those around us. The love, concern and caring that we bring to our relationships have enormous value and worth to us, and to the people we touch. The little things that we do that can't be done by anyone else, other than ourselves, makes us indispensable and of great value. Don't shortchange yourself. Learn to accept this new-found worth, and use it to get the most out of every single day you are alive.

Do yourself a favor. The next time you have your checkbook in your hand, look at the blank check staring you in the face...and imagine putting a dollar value on it for your life AT THAT MOMENT...and remember...

MAKE IT A BIG ONE

Contributed via email by Jason Burt
Original author unknown
THE ROCKS

A WHILE BACK I WAS READING ABOUT AN EXPERT ON SUBJECT OF TIME MANAGEMENT. ONE DAY THIS EXPERT WAS SPEAKING TO A GROUP OF BUSINESS STUDENTS AND, TO DRIVE HOME A POINT, USED AN ILLUSTRATION THOSE STUDENTS WILL NEVER FORGET.

AS THIS MAN STOOD IN FRONT OF THE GROUP OF HIGH-POWERED OVERACHIEVERS HE SAID, "OKAY, TIME FOR A QUIZ." THEN HE PULLED OUT A ONE-GALLON, WIDE-MOUTHED MASON JAR AND SET IT ON A TABLE IN FRONT OF HIM. THEN HE PRODUCED ABOUT A DOZEN FIST-SIZED ROCKS AND CAREFULLY PLACED THEM, ONE AT A TIME,

INTO THE JAR. WHEN THE JAR WAS FILLED TO THE TOP AND NO MORE ROCKS WOULD FIT INSIDE, HE ASKED, "IS THIS JAR FULL?" EVERYONE IN THE CLASS SAID, "YES."

THEN HE SAID, "REALLY?" HE REACHED UNDER THE TABLE AND PULLED OUT A BUCKET OF GRAVEL. THEN HE DUMPED SOME GRAVEL IN AND SHOOK THE JAR CAUSING PIECES OF GRAVEL TO WORK THEMSELVES DOWN INTO THE SPACES BETWEEN THE BIG ROCKS.

THEN HE ASKED THE GROUP ONCE MORE, "IS THE JAR FULL?" BY THIS TIME THE CLASS WAS ONTO HIM. "PROBABLY NOT," ONE OF THEM ANSWERED. "GOOD!" HE REPLIED. HE REACHED UNDER THE TABLE AND BROUGHT OUT A BUCKET OF SAND. HE STARTED DUMPING THE SAND IN AND IT WENT INTO ALL THE SPACES LEFT BETWEEN THE ROCKS AND THE GRAVEL. ONCE MORE HE ASKED THE QUESTION, "IS THIS JAR FULL?" "NO!" THE CLASS SHOUTED.

ONCE AGAIN HE SAID, "GOOD!" THEN HE GRABBED A PITCHER OF WATER AND BEGAN TO POUR IT IN UNTIL THE JAR WAS FILLED TO THE BRIM. THEN HE LOOKED UP AT THE CLASS AND ASKED, "WHAT IS THE POINT OF THIS ILLUSTRATION?"

ONE EAGER BEAVER RAISED HIS HAND AND SAID, "THE POINT IS, NO MATTER HOW FULL YOUR SCHEDULE IS, IF YOU TRY REALLY HARD, YOU CAN ALWAYS FIT SOME MORE THINGS INTO IT!"

"NO," THE SPEAKER REPLIED, "THAT'S NOT THE POINT. THE TRUTH THIS ILLUSTRATION TEACHES US IS: IF YOU DON'T PUT THE BIG ROCKS IN FIRST, YOU'LL NEVER GET THEM IN AT ALL."

WHAT ARE THE 'BIG ROCKS' IN YOUR LIFE? A PROJECT THAT YOU WANT TO ACCOMPLISH? TIME WITH YOUR LOVED ONES? YOUR FAITH, YOUR EDUCATION, YOUR FINANCES? A CAUSE? TEACHING OR MENTORING OTHERS? REMEMBER TO PUT THESE BIG ROCKS IN FIRST OR YOU'LL NEVER GET THEM IN AT ALL.

So, TONIGHT OR IN THE MORNING WHEN YOU ARE RE-
FLECTING ON THIS SHORT STORY, ASK YOURSELF THIS QUES-
TION: WHAT ARE THE 'BIG ROCKS' IN MY LIFE OR BUSI-
NESS? THEN, PUT THOSE IN YOUR JAR FIRST.

CHAPTER 4

My journey through the gauntlet
The 5 phases of grief

A wakening in the hospital room, I.V's in my arm and still attached to the heart monitors, I remember having the strangest dream of dying, and then miraculously coming back to life. As I lay there — staring up at the concerned faces of my wife, friend, nurses, and doctors looking down at me, I realized that what I thought I had dreamed...really did happen.

Over the next days, weeks, months and years, I went through a transformation, a sort of re-birth/new-birth, a changing from who I was to who I was destined to become. I didn't ask for it. I thought I was pretty happy with the person I had gotten so used to being...before my heart attack 'scrambled' up my genes. I went through changes, some overnight, and some that took years to get through successfully. Only recently, through my research, have I discovered that the transformational process or stages that I had gone through were commonly labeled the "five stages of grief." Way back in 1969, Dr. Elisabeth Bubler-Ross wrote, in her book On Death and Dying, that folks go through many situations of change during their lifetime, including the onset of a chronic illness.

According to Dr. Bubler-Ross, each person who goes through the grief stages does so at their own speed. Some deal with each stage at the same pace as the next, while others may go through one stage quickly, and another one extremely slowly. In my case, the one thing that was constant throughout all of my grief stages was that there was no set time limit for how long I dealt with whatever stage of grief I was in at the moment. Some, like denial, took literally years to fully understand, accept, and move through. At times, even though I thought I had handled one of the stages of grief brilliantly, I would back step and have to deal with that stage again, and again, until I finally got it right.

Denial, the first stage that I had to get through, was a real bummer for me. Being a man in my 30's and fairly fit, I could not even imagine that I had landed in the hospital with what I considered to be an "old-age" dilemma. What, a heart attack? "No way" I would say to anyone who could hear me over the commotion in the emergency room of the hospital. I must have eaten something that upset my stomach and gave me indigestion. When I arrived at the hospital deader than a doornail, the emergency room physicians had to bring me back to the living with the "paddles of life", and I was in total and unequivocal denial about the whole episode.

Anger was next on the hit parade. Even if I didn't intentionally express it verbally, I was angry...more at myself than anyone else. I wondered how I could let this happen to me. I would get mad at the dumbest things. The worst part of this was that I was striking out at the people who loved me the most. Looking back on that stage now...I have concluded that I stayed in that stage far longer than I should have.

May I suggest that you read, as I did, the book "Angry all the time - an Emergency Guide to Anger Control" by Ron Potter-Efron, M.S.W. My only regret is that I didn't read that book earlier on. I may have spared myself, my beautiful wife Beth, my kids, and family and friends a lot of anguish.   Even if you have not had a heart attack or chronic illness, but are dealing with being angry, the book will help you understand what anger is, the damage it does to you and the people around you, and how to remove anger from your life once and for all.

Depression wasn't as much a problem to me as it could have been. I have always been an "up" person. Perhaps that is one of the side affects of having a Type-A personality. I did get depressed at times, but the depression didn't last very long. I hid my pain by telling jokes, being funny, and keeping really busy. Only at night did the depression monster creep into the bedroom, attempting to rattle my cage...to no avail. My ego would not allow depression to take hold.

During the Bargaining stage of my recovery from heart disease I would rationalize not taking the medication that I KNEW was there to save my life. Again, my male ego was in denial. I would justify my reasoning by saying..."one day of not exercising, or doing my meditation, or taking my heart medications won't hurt. Right?"

For some people who have developed heart disease, they may start feeling sorry for themselves, and lose hope of conquering the disease. I never needed medication to handle depression, but I would guess that some people might need medical help - if depression becomes all-consuming. I had to remember that this was a stage that needed to be dealt with quickly. I did it, and I know you can, too. Don't let your ego get in the way of asking for and receiving help.

Acceptance was, to me,...the light at the end of the tunnel. I finally accepted that a young man, age 35, happily married, responsible, and loving could, and did, have a near death experience...and lived to tell about it. I honestly believe that I am a better man today, because I

learned that I am not indestructible. I came to fully ac-
knowledge my weaknesses, and started over to build on
my strengths.

Do I still deny having the heart attack? No. Do I get
angry, get depressed, and bargain with myself? Sure I
do, but not as much, or for as long as I have in the past.
Accepting my fate, for what it was, I look at my time in
the hospital as a rebirth, a time to reflect on things the
way I wanted them to be...and then afterwards - a lifetime of "today's" to live in the moment, and make up for
lost time.

SLOW DANCE

© David L. Weatherford
Reprinted with permission

HAVE YOU EVER WATCHED KIDS ON A MERRY-GO-ROUND?
OR LISTENED TO THE RAIN SLAPPING ON THE GROUND?

EVER FOLLOWED A BUTTERFLY'S ERRATIC FLIGHT?
OR GAZED AT THE SUN INTO THE FADING NIGHT?

YOU BETTER SLOW DOWN...DON'T DANCE SO FAST.
TIME IS SHORT. THE MUSIC WON'T LAST.

DO YOU RUN THROUGH EACH DAY ON THE FLY?
WHEN YOU ASK "HOW ARE YOU?" DO YOU HEAR THE RE-
PLY?

WHEN THE DAY IS DONE DO YOU LIE IN YOUR BED
WITH THE NEXT HUNDRED CHORES RUNNING THROUGH
YOUR HEAD?

You'd better slow down...don't dance so fast.
Time is short. The music won't last.

Ever told your child, We'll do it tomorrow?
And in your haste, not see his sorrow?

Ever lost touch, let a good friendship die
Cause you never had time to call and say "Hi?"

You'd better slow down. Don't dance so fast.
Time is short. The music won't last.

When you run so fast to get somewhere
You miss half the fun of getting there.

When you worry and hurry through your day,
It is like an unopened gift....Thrown away.

Life is not a race. Do take it slower
Hear the music before the song is over.

CHAPTER 5

What do you mean, "I'm having a heart attack?"
The Isle of Denial

The Denial phase associated with having "The Big One" is not limited to just the unlucky person that is having a heart attack, or chronic illness. The following story comes from a fellow who was 53 and experiencing his heart attack in bed at about 1 AM. Chuck Daly wrote the following:

"I woke up with really new and different pains in the center of my chest. Although I had never had indigestion in my life, I thought that this might be a possibility, but really didn't think so as my family history dictated that I would die of a heart attack by this age anyway. Within 5 minutes the pains in the left arm started and I was sure that I was having a heart attack and I was ready now to call the paramedics. Unfortunately, I was uncertain as to whether any movement (like reaching for the phone) on my part could promote a final gasp along with my passing into the next life so I decided not to move a muscle and lay as still as possible.

"My next action was to tap my lovely wife on the back-side with the one finger that I dared move. She awoke to tell me that she was kind of tired, but I explained instead that I was certain that I was having a heart attack. To my surprise she protested this statement like she was in a position to know better than me. All of a sudden, I realized that

she was in Denial instead of me and I enjoyed a brief moment of deathbed humor before I realized that.

"I was the person in the deathbed. I remained still and calm; again not wanting to move less I hasten my departure from this earth. I assertively vocalized my position that I was certain that I was having a heart attack and insisted that she call 911. She then jumped out of bed, flipped on the bathroom light and disappeared into that doorless room maintaining atypical "submarine under siege" silence. As the phone was on the other side of the bedroom away from the bathroom, I began to wonder what she was doing in there for so long. Being both an engineer and statistician I began to calibrate the amount of movement to my head that I might risk to look into the bathroom and maybe get a bounced view of her in the mirror to see what she was doing in there.

"I then began the death defying micro movements of my head as I was now curious enough to risk death just to answer the burning question in my mind. After completing the head movements and enjoying a moment of success in still being alive, I must have popped my eyes open to the max as I saw that she was leaning forward into the mirror applying the last bit of makeup to her face.

"Needless to say, I encouraged her to finish her task after she called 911 and finally she complied. I was subsequently saved by the paramedics and doctors who used modern techniques to give me the opportunity to be here today telling you this story of Denial, not by me, but by the support personnel that you might incorrectly assume would not retard the process of your survival. As they say... "All is Well That Ends Well", but I still chuckle at the events of that very scary evening."

When I was going through my denial, finding myself talking about the future was not uncommon. Talking only about the future, and avoiding the present with all the hurt, pain, and confusion, was all I could handle at the time. After the actual heart attack happened, I would avoid discussing how I felt. It wasn't that I didn't want to talk to anyone, but I couldn't put what my body and soul was going through into words that non-survivors could fully understand. Denial was a buffer against what I was going through. My isolation and denial of what happened was my way of learning how to cope with what happened to me.

I learned some valuable tricks to maneuvering through this phase of my grief and pain. Of utmost importance was to be nonjudgmental of the way that my friends and family dealt with my new illness. I saw what was in their hearts and it was good. Early on, I took full responsibility for my illness, and my fast recovery. Not taking things personally was a hard lesson to learn. I kept saying "why me?" Lastly, I learned to talk again, and to listen to the wonderful advice that my family and friends gave me. Being an action-oriented type individual, I attempted to move through this stage of grief and loss quickly. There were times that I felt I completely conquered this stage, but from time to time, slipped back into it for no reason at all. Only after I fully accepted this stage, in both my mind and my heart, and that denying what happened only hurt myself, and those around me, did I fully recover from this phase of grief and loss.

Like Chuck's wonderful story of his wife's denial of his heart problem, we all work through it in our own way, and at our own speed.

Being asked one day what was the surest way of remaining happy in this world, the Emperor Sigismund of Germany replied: "Only do in health what you have promised to do when you are sick."

– Anon –

CHAPTER 6

Anger Management
"Anger" is only one letter from "danger"

After the tragedy of the attacks on the world trade center in New York, the news media from around the world started to quote President George W. Bush's proclamation that there is a "quiet, unyielding anger" toward the terrorists. The Wednesday after that terrible event, I was at a restaurant in Thousand Oaks, California, having lunch with a friend, and as I entered the eating establishment, I looked upon the faces of the people there and saw pure rage, bewilderment, depression, and anger.

Everyone was angry.

The faces of the people in the eatery were as red as a Washington "red delicious" apple. Being a regular there, and very interested in what the people had to say and feel about the attacks, I proceeded to do a "man on the street" interview of the folks. The remarks, though not unexpected...were however, nonetheless, shocking. I asked the same question of everyone in the eating establishment, which was "Being as angry as you are right now...what will it take to get you to move on and calm down and get on with your life?" Every person interviewed was angry...almost to the point of not being about to speak about it. One person whom I had never seen before was far more contemplative than the rest. After sitting there for the longest time, he put his glass of iced tea down on the table, looked up at me and slowly and angrily stated he wanted to leave the restaurant, buy a weapon and kill someone. I was so shocked by this I asked him "who" he wanted to kill, and he stated without hesitation - "anyone." Being so enraged, he could not distinguish between the terrorists, and "anyone else." This was not an isolated case. Everyone had the same instant rage...and in most cases, were so angry that they couldn't even talk about it.

When I had my heart attack, I remember two things that went through my mind at the time. I was scared, and I was angry. Looking back, I, too, had a quiet, unyielding anger. Not at anyone in particular, but mostly at myself for allowing this heart attack to happen. I realized years later that the anger was misplaced and totally not realistic.

What could I have done then...and what can people do now to manage rage and anger? The following may help.

Control the direction of your anger

The people in the restaurant were misdirecting their rage to innocent bystanders who had nothing to do with what happened thousands of miles away. Don't take your anger out on "innocents." One of our friends is from India, but people have already started to look at her as though she was from the part of the world where the U.S. government believed the terrorists were from. Because she didn't want to be singled out, she began acting as though she were of Hispanic descent, thus hopefully protecting herself from this misguided anger people have displaced. If you are angry with someone, talk to them about it...and don't misdirect your feelings toward someone else...just because they are in the line of fire, or are convenient.

Disengage from the anger

Try not to be part of the anger, take a deep breath, and pull back, looking at the event as if you were a bystander. By briefly disengaging from the anger event, just for a moment, you might get a better perspective on what is really happening around you. By not becoming reactionary, you will have a better handle on the ultimate outcome of the event by controlling your own actions wisely.

Use each other for support

With my heart attack, as well as my feelings toward the terrorists, and learning from many years studying the consequences of misdirected anger, I have learned to lean on and trust my family, friends, and sometimes, total strangers when I need to "vent" and discuss my issues and feelings surrounding anger. For a guy, you might find that very hard to do, if not almost impossible (at first), but trusting and asking for support is critical to releasing the anger stressors you are feeling.

Talk about anger to family and friends

We all get angry. How we handle that anger makes us different from all the creatures in the animal world. Accept the fact that EVERYONE gets angry from time to time. My wife would listen to me for hours while I vented my anger. She knew that I was not angry with her, but I just needed to get stuff off my chest. Her care, compassion, and concern, while listening, and without criticism and judgment, worked miracles.

Don't become animals

There are two things animals know how to do really well, and that's "Fight or Flee." Don't become an animal if you are mad or angry. One moment of anger can kill you...literally. If you get so angry you start seeing red, you are about to go into meltdown. Most likely your blood pressure is going through the roof, your blood vessels are not getting enough blood circulating, and more importantly, your brain is not getting the necessary oxygen to function and think clearly. Learn to RELAX.

Be careful not to offend

I find that when I get mad, I may inadvertently offend the very person that can help me the most, and that's my wife, and best friend. Guys, if you piss off your wife, or significant other, just toss your toothbrush in your overnight bag and proceed quickly to the doghouse. Don't bite the hand that feeds you - in this case it's the one person that loves you unconditionally and cares enough to listen to your rantings and ravings, and after its all said and done, says "I love you."

Let your emotions cool down

One secret I have learned is to let my emotions cool down before I say anything that may get me into trouble. Think of it as the "Jack-in-the-box" we all had when we were children. I used to have one when I was a kid. Once I opened the top of the box, and the Jack-in-the-box popped out, I could not figure out how to get him back in the box. The same thing goes with saying things in the heat of anger. Once you say something...you can NEVER take it back. Things said in anger have started wars, caused divorces, and have gotten good people fired from jobs. Be careful what you say. Remember, let your emotions cool WAY down before you say anything that may get you into trouble.

Being more in control means being less in Anger

I like to watch shows that have actors using the martial arts to defend the innocent and win the day. I have done a little martial arts in my day, and, always marveled at the "Black Belt" masters that have trained themselves to be cool under fire. While surrounded by two or three aggressors, the Black Belt martial artist will skillfully, and masterfully, defend his or her turf without mussing a hair on his/her head. It seems that the more they are in control, the more out of control the opponent is.

Congratulate yourself when you win over Anger

We humans tend to focus on too much negativity. If something goes wrong, we blame ourselves. I have been known to say, "if I had only been a better negotiator, I could have won that argument" on more than one occasion. Sometimes we buy into the irrational belief that we can do everything right...all the time. Remember, we are human. We make mistakes, we get mad, and we get angry. We also learn from our trials and tribulations and strive to constantly improve ourselves. Be sure to congratulate yourself on your accomplishments - when you win over an anger episode by being calm and rational. Relish in the warmth of your success. Take time to really savor how it feels to control and conquer your anger. Learn to forgive yourself when you get angry or mad. Use this as a yardstick on how you are doing toward moving toward your goal of an anger-free existence.

Other ways to handle and dissipate anger when it appears:

* Set a timeline to be angry and don't exceed it.
* If you are angry with someone, tell him or her how you are feeling - but that you still love them.
* Learn the technique of "I feel, I want, I need."

An example of this would be "I feel that what you did was unjust. I want to explain my side of the story and I need you to please sit there and listen to me without judging me."

* Learn Conflict resolution techniques.
* Write a letter telling that person you are angry or mad with them...but don't mail it. Sometimes just taking action will help you deal with the anger you feel. On many occasions, I have been so angry, that I literally see "red", but I know that once I say something, I can NEVER take it back. I do write the letter, but I then either let it sit on my desk for a day or so...or I toss it in my shredder. As the teeth of the shredder cut the document to pieces, I visualize my anger dissipating.
* Write a letter telling that person you are angry or mad with them...and mail it...but wait two days after you have written it to send it to them. Giving you time to reflect, edit, correct, modify, or add/delete sections makes the letter more affective than sending it while you are enraged. The same thing holds true with sending a letter via email. We are now in a world of instant messaging, and sometimes the ability to react instantly may come back to bite you. The added downside to sending an email while angry, is that there now is a hard copy record of what you said that can and usually is used against the sender at a later date.
* Try to see the argument from THEIR point of view.

Don't buy into the concept that the more anger you display, the more in control you are, because it's just not true. Just the opposite actually is happening. You are less in control. Stay in control. Being more in control means less in Anger.

♥   ♥   ♥

The man who makes everything that leads to happiness
depend upon himself, and not upon other men,
has adopted the very best plan for living happily.

– Plato –

CHAPTER 7

Learn to conquer road rage
"5 minutes ago, the person in the other car
was a really nice guy"

Road rage. It's all over the evening news. Special shows now on all the major TV channels highlight police chases through the streets of the city worldwide...with the outcome usually having the perpetrator smashing his or her car into a building, another parked car, or flipping their car over and ending up in a ball of flames at the bottom of a ditch. The media has made it very clear that road rage is very much alive and well. Have you ever been mad while behind the wheel of your car? Don't kid yourselves, we all have. But why worry about road rage? What possible impact could it have on your physical well-being?

What's the big deal about a little road rage? Everyone gets mad at other drivers from time to time. Sure. We all do! It's how we handle the situation that either gets us into trouble, or keeps us calm, composed, and under control while driving our car on the road.

What are the physical ramifications of not controlling your impulses, and developing road rage? The ultimate question we should be asking is this: Can out-of-control anger trigger a heart attack? In a report in the prestigious medical journal Circulation, 1600 people were interviewed by the scientists a few days after they had heart attacks to determine their level of anger before they were

stricken. The results confirmed a direct correlation between anger and heart disease. The scientists found anger doubled the risk of a heart attack in the two hours
that followed the outbreak. But why? According to the
report, anger triggered an immediate increase in blood
pressure, and heart rate, which in turn, caused choles-
terol-laden plaque to break free of the artery walls. Once
the plaque had broken free, it developed into clots, which
in turn blocked the flow of blood.

How do I handle road rage? Well, the first thing I do is
leave my male EGO outside the car door. I also realize
that the car I am driving is a lethal weapon if I choose to
use it that way. Even If I am alone, I visualize myself
driving some of the people I love the most, (my wife,
kids, grandkids, parents, or friends) in the back seat...and
I would never put them in harm's way.

Change your attitude toward what is happening to
YOU. Instead of thinking about WHY ME — ...think —
WHY HIM/HER. Why is this happening to them? What
is their intent for what we think is irrational behavior? I
know that when I had my heart attack, I can only presume that my wife would have broken every traffic law
on the books to get me to the nearest hospital in time to
save my life. To a casual observer, however, it might have
been seen as someone who was in a very big hurry to get
somewhere, and thus could have developed road rage in
a big way. To my wife, she was trying to save my life, but
to someone else in the car next to her, they perceived a
raging maniac who had no idea what was happening.
Same event...but with two different intents, and two different points-of-view.

It really has to do with leaving your EGO at the car
door, and not imposing your pre-defined judgment on
what you think is actually causing the other driver to
drive and act so erratically.

If someone cuts in front of me, I now instinctively take my foot off the accelerator, just for a moment. It doesn't affect the speed of the car...but does affect my view of the situation. I am taking a "time-out." It doesn't slow the car down too much, but more importantly, it forces me to "slow down" mentally - just for a moment. I believe it disengages the mental from the physical. Sometimes we do things in automatic mode without really thinking about the consequences, and by taking my foot off the gas...just for a moment, I have broken this autopilot. I then take a deep breath, and wonder why they are in such a big hurry. Is there a pregnant lady laid out in the back seat, out of view? Has the person in the car just heard that his child or family member is sick and he/she needs to get to them as soon as possible? Perhaps by me backing off, allowing the person to pass by me, I am in some way helping them with their problem. Maybe not...but at least I stay in control.

Other things that can be done to prevent being attacked by the Road Rage Warrior:

* Stay in the car. Don't run the car off the road, get out and pounce on the driver. He or she may be bigger, meaner and or nastier than you expect.
* Don't flip the Road Rage Warrior the finger, or any other offensive gesture.
* Say you are sorry - even if you know you are right, and don't mean it. It won't help if you are dead right - you are still dead, and they are still driving. You can either mouth the words "Sorry" or better yet, make a SORRY sign and flash it at them through the window. According to the U.S. Highway Safety Office, 85 percent of the road ragers said that they would drop the matter if the other "careless" driver just apologized. Most of the road

ragers were so surprised that someone would show a sign, and say they were sorry, that they smiled and drove off.

* Don't take the problems on the road personally.
* Avoid eye contact with an aggressive driver, and don't tailgate.
* Use your horn very sparingly. The honk usually is a trigger for the aggressive driver to act nastily.
* Act like the other person in the car is your best friend, and assume they feel the same way. Perception is everything.

Remember, there are hundreds of reasons why the person cut you off...and you know none of them. The only thing you know is that by being calm, staying cool, and relaxed, you stay IN-CONTROL, your blood pressure hasn't risen, and you get to your destination in one piece. Think about it.

♥   ♥   ♥

Good advice, for the guys out there
A guy in traffic
Author: Unknown

I WAS RIDING TO WORK YESTERDAY WHEN I OBSERVED A FEMALE DRIVER CUT RIGHT IN FRONT OF A PICKUP TRUCK CAUSING HIM TO HAVE TO DRIVE ON TO THE SHOULDER. THIS EVIDENTLY PISSED THE DRIVER OFF ENOUGH THAT HE HUNG HIS HEAD OUT HIS WINDOW AND FLIPPED THE WOMAN OFF.

"MAN, THAT GUY IS STUPID" I THOUGHT TO MYSELF. I ALWAYS SMILE NICELY AND WAVE IN A SHEEPISH MANNER WHENEVER A FEMALE DOES ANYTHING TO ME IN TRAFFIC AND HERE'S WHY:

I DRIVE 38 MILES EACH WAY EVERY DAY TO WORK, THAT'S 76 MILES. OF THESE, 16 MILES EACH WAY IS BUMPER-TO-BUMPER. MOST OF THE BUMPER-TO-BUMPER IS ON AN 8-LANE HIGHWAY SO IF YOU JUST LOOK AT THE 7 LANES I AM NOT IN, THAT MEANS I PASS SOMETHING LIKE A NEW CAR EVERY 40 FEET PER LANE. THAT'S 7 CARS EVERY 40 FEET FOR 32 MILES.

THAT WORKS OUT TO BE 982 CARS EVERY MILE, OR 31,424 CARS.

EVEN THOUGH THE REST OF THE 34 MILES IS NOT BUMPER-TO-BUMPER. I FIGURE I PASS AT LEAST ANOTHER 4000 CARS. THAT BRINGS THE NUMBER TO SOMETHING LIKE 36,000 CARS I PASS EVERY DAY. STATISTICALLY HALF OF THESE ARE DRIVEN BY A FEMALE, THAT'S 18,000.

IN ANY GIVEN GROUP OF FEMALES 1 IN 28 ARE HAVING THE WORST DAY OF THEIR PERIOD. THAT'S 642. ACCORDING TO COSMOPOLITAN, 70% DESCRIBE THEIR LOVE LIFE AS DISSATISFYING OR UNREWARDING, THAT'S 449. ACCORDING TO THE NATIONAL INSTITUTES OF HEALTH, 22% OF ALL FEMALES HAVE SERIOUSLY CONSIDERED SUICIDE OR HOMICIDE, THAT'S 98. AND 34% DESCRIBE MEN AS THEIR BIGGEST PROBLEM, THAT'S 33.

ACCORDING TO THE NATIONAL RIFLE ASSOCIATION 5% OF ALL FEMALES CARRY WEAPONS AND THIS NUMBER IS INCREASING. THAT MEANS THAT EVERY SINGLE DAY, I DRIVE PAST AT LEAST ONE FEMALE THAT HAS A LOUSY LOVE LIFE, THINKS MEN ARE HER BIGGEST PROBLEM, HAS SERIOUSLY CONSIDERED SUICIDE OR HOMICIDE, IS HAVING THE WORST DAY OF HER PERIOD, AND IS ARMED.

NO MATTER WHAT SHE DOES IN TRAFFIC, I WOULDN'T DREAM OF FLIPPING HER OFF.

CHAPTER 8

Angry words make for a hurt'n heart
Words that Heal

Dale Carnegie said once "Act enthusiastically, and you'll be enthusiastic." Horace Rutledge was quoted as stating "When you look at the world in a narrow way, how narrow it seems! When you look at it in a mean way, how mean it is! When you look at it selfishly, how selfish it is! But when you look at it in a broad, generous friendly spirit, what wonderful people you find in it." And finally, James E. Sweeney said "You can promote your healing by your thinking."

"When people asked, I used to tell them how sick I was. The more I talked about being sick, the worse I got. I started saying, 'I'm getting better.' It took a while, but then I started to feel better, too."
– Michael Hirsch, person with AIDs –

"Some patients I see are actually draining into their bodies the diseased thoughts of their minds." – Zachary T. Bercovitz, M.D.

How many times have we been around parents of children and overheard them say something like "watch your mouth, young lady", or "don't say that...you'll hurt their feelings?" At one time or another, we all have inadvertently been in a position to hear conversations between parent and child.

Looking back at my life, I can remember when words spoken by another have inflicted untold physical, as well as mental, distress upon my body, soul, and spirit. I have been brought to anger by the mean use of words bestowed upon me by friend, family, or foe. Think back into your past and see if you were affected by criticism, untrue blame, being called a hurtful nickname, or a victim of unwarranted and malicious gossip. Remember how it affected you at the moment of occurrence, as well as the length of time it took for you to get over it.There is a company that sells a series of cassette tapes teaching folks how to increase their vocabulary...by listening to audio-tapes. The company spokesman states that by using words correctly, you can increase your status in your business life, your position on the social and economic ladder, by having a better command of the English language.

All these people understood the importance of word usage...both from the point of view of hurting people's feelings to that of healing physical and mental ailments, as well as increasing your economic value to society and your family. As in the example above with the parent disciplining the child, or the AIDs patient who fully understands that words can either hinder or heal, we all can learn to use words more effectively and efficiently, to heal what is ailing us, to comfort ourselves, or those around us, or move a business project or task along to a successful conclusion.

Experiment No. 1: Try this. Wherever you are right now, if there are people around you, listen to the words they use and the reactions by the people those words are addressed to - who hear those words. Is the reaction positive or negative? Is the reaction a weak one, or a strong one? How do you react by hearing those words...knowing you are not involved with those people at all? Go to a mall, or a shopping center, sit quietly, and jot down all the words you hear. On a piece of paper, draw a line down the middle of the paper, and one across the top from left to right. On the left side, write the words "negative/hurtful", and on the right side of the paper write the words "positive/healing." While sitting there, place the words you hear in either the left or right column based on them either being negative/hurtful, or positive/healing. It shouldn't take you too long to notice a pattern of how people are talking to each other, and how you are reacting to those conversations.

Experiment No.2: This may be a little hard to do without practice, but after a few minutes, you will get the hang of it. While talking to other people, listen to the words YOU use. Are they negative, stressful, or hurtful in any way? Or are they positive, healing and encouraging words? Remember the first exercise, and how you reacted to "other" people's words. If you are using negative words, are you getting negative feedback from the person who you are chatting with? After doing the second exercise for a day or so, you will start to understand your "standard operating procedure" in relation to talking to others.

We all "self talk" to ourselves. Even when we are talking to other people, our mind is talking. Our subconscious mind is always chatting. It's our nature. We can't turn it off. We were born that way. I was watching TV the other day and came across a great illustration. A guy was trying to make a decision on something. Standing on his left and right shoulders were a couple of little women about two inches tall. One had a devilish mannerism and the other was angelic in nature. The advertisers wanted us to believe that the two little people were the personification of his mother's good and bad consciences trying to control his behavior. As he tried to make a decision on his own, the good and bad consciences were battling to have the final say in how this young man acted. We all act that way. What comes out after the battle is over are words that outwardly display which one of our consciences won. If we use angry, condescending, vile or hurtful words, then we know which side of our conscience won that particular engagement. On the other hand, if encouraging, healing and/or loving words are spoken by us, we then can tell who triumphed in that engagement.

Experiment No. 3: We have the ability to train ourselves to self-talk or verbally express things in a positive manner. Using the same list format as the first two experiments above, list the words YOU are using when you self talk or talk out loud. Are they positive or negative, hurtful, or healing? Harming or helping? Look at the list of negative words and substitute positive words in their place. Practice saying the same negative statement, in a positive way.

I remember when I was laid up in the hospital, my old boss called, and the hospital put him through to my bedside phone. I picked up the phone, and immediately knew that the call was not "helpful and healing" in any way. My boss didn't care one iota how I was feeling. He didn't call to see if there was anything he, or the office staff, could do for me while I was in the hospital.

He wanted to know "why" I missed the regional sales meeting, where the end of month sales figures were, and had I booked the flight for both he and I to Denver, Colorado, for a conference we were to attend the next weekend. His words were cruel, hurtful, and harmful, and the blood pressure monitor reflected the stress I was feeling because of the words he was saying, and my reaction to those words. After listening to his conversation, I made a snap decision that changed the course of my life forever. I told him that the problem I was having was a result of his poor management, and I then quit my job...right then and there. Because I was still attached to the heart and blood pressure monitors, I watched in amazement as my blood pressure dropped 20 points within seconds after I made my decision. Because I took control of the words I used, I am alive today to talk about it, and learn from it.

From that moment on...every morning when I arise, I say to myself "Every day...in every way, I am getting better and better." I try to do "positive self talk" as much as I can. I listen to my words as I say them, and try to put a positive spin on my conversation whenever humanly possible, and I do listen to other people when they chat with each other and listen to the words they use. I try to use words that encourage, add hope, provide guidance, mentor and heal. Do I falter? Sure. That's what makes us human. But I realize that fact and go on to enjoy this fantastic, marvelous life...knowing I am getting better and better, every day in every way.

Temper
Author unknown

WHEN I HAVE LOST MY TEMPER I HAVE LOST MY
REASON, TOO.
I'M NEVER PROUD OF ANYTHING WHICH ANGRILY I DO.

WHEN I HAVE TALKED IN ANGER AND MY CHEEKS WERE
FLAMING RED,
I HAVE ALWAYS UTTERED SOMETHING WHICH I WISH I
HADN'T SAID.

IN ANGER I HAVE NEVER DONE A KINDLY DEED OR WISE,
BUT MANY THINGS FOR WHICH I FELT I SHOULD
APOLOGIZE.

IN LOOKING BACK ACROSS MY LIFE, AND ALL I'VE LOST
    OR MADE,
I CAN'T RECALL A SINGLE TIME WHEN FURY EVER PAID.

SO I STRUGGLE TO BE PATIENT, FOR I'VE REACHED A
    WISER AGE;
I DO NOT WANT TO DO A THING OR SPEAK A WORD IN RAGE.

I HAVE LEARNED BY SAD EXPERIENCE THAT WHEN MY
    TEMPER FLIES,
I NEVER DO A WORTHY THING, A DECENT DEED OR WISE.

CHAPTER 9

"Man, I'm depressed"

"M an, I'm depressed" was heard throughout the hall way of the Cardiac Care Unit at Saint Johns Medical Clinic, in Oxnard, California. As the nurses rushed into the hospital room to see what the commotion was all about, the young man was trying to un-tie the gown that was placed on him when he arrived in the ER the night before. The young man didn't really have a choice of clothing to wear, mind you. He was there because his heart had failed on the way to the hospital, and should have been thankful that he had clothes on at all. Rushing to his side, the nurse asked frantically "what's the matter young man?" He then said, "Is this the only style and color gown there is?"

We all get depressed sometimes, and how we handle it makes us individuals. We can't be happy all the time, now can we? When a national tragedy occurs, such as when the President of the United States was assassinated, or there is a tragedy like in New York City and the Pentagon, in September, 2001, the whole country, and the world, becomes depressed.

Over time, however, we overcome our depression, move on with the daily routine we call living, and through it all, we grow from the experience to become a better person. Grieving for the loss of a loved one, or realizing the loss of a freedom (our own lifestyle as a result of a chronic illness) we'd taken for granted, can be a depressing time in one's life. Everyone handles depression in their own way - in the case of the young man in the hospital, he used humor to defray his depression, panic, being scared, and almost losing his life to heart disease.

Psychologists say that being depressed is the freezing of one's emotion in time. Until one moves through this phase of their life, they cannot and will not get, or feel, better about themselves and the world around them.

What are the symptoms of depression? Withdrawal from the normal routines of living; becoming isolated from the people one interacts with on a daily basis; stopping the activities that one routinely does; having suicidal thoughts and intentions; feeling guilt about an event or an action; eating or drinking in excess; having a loss of normal sleep patterns; being restless (more than normal for your personality); having a loss of concentration; hopelessness and helplessness; being uninterested in sex, eating, or having "fun"; being bored, apathetic, and being more tired than normal. Basically being depressed is having a lack of self-esteem and showing no interest in the world around you.

So, what is the cure for depression? The first thing I would like to point out is that if you have had suicidal thoughts, then you need to get treatment immediately. Talk to someone, or call the Suicide Hotline in your area. Remember, you are not the first person that got depressed, and will not be the last, so rest assured you are not alone. The important thing here is to seek guidance. People do care.

❤ ❤ ❤

Learn as if you were going to live forever;
Live as if you were going to die tomorrow
- Anon -

The following may help you get "through" this time of depression:

* Read the comic section in your local newspaper.
* Hang around someone who can give you a little Love'n.
* Take action and keep on keeping on.
* Act enthusiastic and you'll be enthusiastic. In other words, force yourself to be happy. It may feel like it's a phony feeling, but do it long enough, and it becomes contagious.
* Meditate and visualize yourself in a happy, non-depressed mood.
* Get physical. Go out for a walk, chase your significant other around the bed, chase the dog for a change, instead of having the dog chase you.
* Get more facts - if you are depressed about some "thing" then find out all you can about it. The more you know, the less you will be depressed about it. Knowledge is power.
* Get more sleep.
* Hang around happy people. Go see a comedy at the movie. Read a funny joke on the Internet.
* Make a habit of smiling 10 times per day. I never knew anyone that could smile and be depressed at the same time.
* Eat comfort food. Think about the times you were happy and what food you ate during that time. Where do you think Chicken Soup came from? Some grandmother back in history tried to cheer up someone in her family by feeding them chicken soup, and it worked then, so it will work now.
* Be an optimist - just for the day. Fake it if you have to. It might become a habit.

* Accept that you are depressed, and then give yourself a set amount of time to feel that way - say an hour. Once the hour is up, force yourself to be happy and be done with it.
* Start to recognize the signs that your depression is ending.
* Learn to improve communications in your personal and professional life.

As someone said, "this too will pass." Being depressed is part of who we are, but staying depressed in not healthy for us, or our loved ones. Work through it, talk about it to your loved ones, and move on.

The value of time
Author unknown

To realize the value of one year: Ask a student who has failed a final exam.

To realize the value of one month: Ask a mother who has given birth to a premature baby.

To realize the value of one week: Ask an editor of a weekly newspaper.

To realize the value of one hour: Ask the lovers who are waiting to meet.

To realize the value of one minute: Ask the person who has missed the train, bus or plane.

To realize the value of one second: Ask a person who has survived an accident.

To realize the value of one millisecond: Ask the person who has won a silver medal in the Olympics.

Time waits for no one.

Treasure every moment you have. You will treasure it even more when you can share it with someone special.

CHAPTER 10

You mean "I can have sex?"
It's ok to "Saddle UP"

I know what you're thinking. When you picked this book up at the bookstore, glancing at the chapter titles (as we all do before we spend good money on a book), you came across this chapter title, and said...WOW. He's talking about SEX. How bold, brash, and absolutely taboo to talk about a subject like this in book like this one.

Remember, this book was written as a survival guide...and as a guy...you have to get the subject of sex into the book or it just won't sell.

After my bout with heart disease happened, and I returned to what I consider to be a normal life, there was a little bit of residue left over because of the experience. There were times when I was afraid to make love to the most wonderful, beautiful women in the world...my wife. I was fearful that my lovemaking would cause me to have another heart attack. Let me repeat the last statement, because it is extremely important to understand that I, and probably you...were afraid to make love to your partner because of fear of a repeat occurrence of heart attack.

According to a number of journal articles from the American Journal of Cardiology over the last few years, it is "extraordinarily safe" for most men with heart disease to enter into lovemaking. I would like to state, for the record, that I am not a medical doctor, and am not giving medical advice. Instead, being a male of sound body and mind, I had to deal with this issue early on after my attack. You should always consult your own medical practitioner on this matter...to be on the safe side. From information in these reports, men, on average, made love only half as often as they did before the attack. The reason was not that there was a problem with the heart muscle, but because these men were "afraid" that by having sex, they would have another heart attack. In a University of Toronto study, less than 12 percent of heart attack survivors had chest pain after love making, versus 36 percent while riding a stationary bicycle. Another study states that the absolute risk for a heart attack during the lovemaking activity for men, who have had a heart attack, is 2 chances per million...per hour in men that are healthy and middle-aged. Even in "high-risk" cases where the patients with ischemic heart disease participated in lovemaking, the heart attacks were 20 chances per million per hour. According to one study, in most cases, the heart rate rose only 4-8 beats per minute.

I would like to point out that the act of lovemaking does not necessitate people being in great physical shape. One study stated that if you can comfortably walk up two flights of stairs without getting out of breath, you could most likely make love.

During my research for this chapter, I came across some interesting facts. Staying with your regular partner is the best way of preventing a heart attack during lovemaking. In an Emery Medical School study on the subject, men's pulse rates never went higher than 100 beats per minute and the heart rate was normal in men who made love to their wives. On the other hand, when a mistress was involved with the man's lovemaking escapades, the heart beat irregularly 130 times a minute or more. Even a Japanese Journal of Legal Medicine study indicated that 80% of men (or more) who died during sex were not making whoopie with their wives. The last bit of information on the subject is from the famous heart researcher from the University of Pennsylvania, David Kritchevsky, who wrote:

> Heart beats stay at normal rate,
> When one beds down with legal mate.
> But roosting in another's nest,
> flirts with cardiac arrest

I did not have the medical proof that making love probably would not harm me 15 years ago. I had to deal with it alone. Thank god for my loving wife, Beth, for understanding what I was going through and being patient with me. The world has changed in the last 15 years, and there is the Internet, and lots of information readily available to you on this subject. Talk to your partner, and/or your doctor about what you are going through. Don't lose the intimacy with the one person who loves you the most.

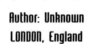

Author: Unknown
LONDON, England

ALL OF LONDON WAS ABUZZ RECENTLY WHEN NINE RESIDENTS OF THE EDITH SCARBOROUGH NURSING HOME WERE TOLD THAT THEY MUST FIND A NEW PLACE TO LIVE AFTER THEY ATTEMPTED A LATE-NIGHT ORGY. THAT'S RIGHT, THEY WERE CAUGHT IN THE RECREATION ROOM ATTEMPTING TO HAVE A SEX PARTY TO THE EXOTIC SOUNDS OF THE RUMBA MUSIC. THEIR AGES RANGED FROM 78 TO 95.

THE BRITISH MEDICAL JOURNAL SAYS THAT MEN WHO HAVE A SEXUAL ORGASM TWO TIMES OR MORE A WEEK HAVE 1/2 THE RISK OF DEATH OF THOSE THAT DON'T.

C H A P T E R 11

Recognizing the type of personality you were born with

During my childhood, I watched my father go off to work every day and...more times than I can remember, he worked late into the evenings...coming home late from whatever job he was paid to do at the time. He had a strong work ethic, a dedication to getting the job done, and done well, and was a wonderful provider for the family. Like most young men, I watched how my dad dealt with life's issues, and I took away from those observations my own sense of how I should live my life. Dad seemed to be able to control every aspect of his life with ease, dealing with every eventuality with finesse.

Eventually growing into manhood, and venturing out on my own, I attempted to take away what I had learned from him, and developed my own sense of how to deal with life's trials and tribulations in a way I could handle as easily as my dad did. Man - was I mistaken!

I was always an active kid growing up. Being restless had become the norm for me. For example, while I was in the school library, working on an assignment, other kids could sit quietly reading. I, on the other hand, was tapping my fingers, or feet, while humming a song or two, chewing gum, and day dreaming... all at the same time. My mother recently told me that I was so restless and uncontrollable when I was very young, that the school had no other way of dealing with me than to force me to sit in the hallway for the first two years of my education.

We are taught that as we grow up, we mature, and as part of this maturity, some of our childlike mannerisms fall away. We become adults, with all the rights and privileges therein. I look back on the time just before my heart attack and realize that I had learned to mask a lot of my hyperactive behavior that I carried with me from childhood. I really thought I had learned to control the monster within me to the point that no one would find out that the monster had followed me through time...and now was very much alive in my adulthood.

One of the traits that I learned to live with was trying to do more than two things at a time. For example, in my younger days, I would read a magazine...while at the same time watching the news on TV. Or, I would work on something, while talking on the telephone. Waiting in line was like going to the dentist and getting a tooth extracted. Actually, that would have been easier for me than waiting in line.

Even today, my wife says that I eat - no...inhale my food - faster than anyone she knows. She, on the other hand, savors her food. For the longest time, I would over schedule myself with "busy" work. Being in the sales business at the time, I thought that was the normal thing to do.

I had a problem sitting still and doing nothing for any length of time. For example, I was extremely impatient with people in the service industry. On more than one occasion, I would pester the waiters when my food wasn't ready quickly enough...to a level of embarrassment.

I think the biggest issue I had before my heart attack was that I had difficulty accepting criticism from anyone. There were times that I would have revenge fantasies toward the person who gave the criticism. Today, I am happy to say...I've been able to see criticism for what it truly is...a way for me to grow and learn.

Through my research, I have come to discover that I had the classic symptoms of what Dr. Meyer Friedman, M.D, cardiologist, in 1959 termed as having a Type-A personality. Knowing that I could now put a name to the monster that had followed me through the decades was comforting. I could now put my arms around it, wrestle it to the ground, and whip it to within an inch of its life.

But so what? In a nutshell: Because I had all the symptoms of a Type A personality, and if I didn't change my ways, and fast, I had two to three times more likely a chance for a second heart attack, or sudden death, than my Type-B brethren.

So what is this Type-B personality that we all should strive to become...and where can I buy some? The Type-A personality seems to run in my family, as well as being heavily promoted in American society. The question I started to ask was - is there any way to reduce the negative effects of stress? Could I become a Type-B personality? Could I go from a driven, competitive soul to an easy-going, laid back person...and relax? Read on and find out the secret.

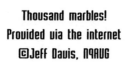

Thousand marbles!
Provided via the internet
©Jeff Davis, N9AUG

THE OLDER I GET, THE MORE I ENJOY SATURDAY MORNINGS. PERHAPS IT'S THE QUIET SOLITUDE THAT COMES WITH BEING THE FIRST TO RISE, OR MAYBE IT'S THE UNBOUNDED JOY OF NOT HAVING TO BE AT WORK. EITHER WAY, THE FIRST FEW HOURS OF A SATURDAY MORNING ARE MOST ENJOYABLE.

A FEW WEEKS AGO, I WAS SHUFFLING TOWARD THE BASE-
MENT STAIRS WITH A STEAMING CUP OF COFFEE IN ONE
HAND AND THE MORNING PAPER IN THE OTHER. WHAT
BEGAN AS A TYPICAL SATURDAY MORNING, TURNED INTO
ONE OF THOSE LESSONS THAT LIFE SEEMS TO HAND YOU
FROM TIME TO TIME.

LET ME TELL YOU ABOUT IT.

I TURNED THE DIAL UP INTO THE PHONE PORTION OF
THE BAND ON MY HAM RADIO IN ORDER TO LISTEN TO A
SATURDAY MORNING SWAP NET. ALONG THE WAY, I CAME
ACROSS AN OLDER SOUNDING CHAP, WITH A TREMENDOUS
SIGNAL AND A GOLDEN VOICE. YOU KNOW THE KIND, HE
SOUNDED LIKE HE SHOULD BE IN THE BROADCASTING BUSI-
NESS. HE WAS TELLING WHOEVER HE WAS TALKING WITH
SOMETHING ABOUT "A THOUSAND MARBLES."

I WAS INTRIGUED AND STOPPED TO LISTEN TO WHAT HE
HAD TO SAY. "WELL, TOM, IT SURE SOUNDS LIKE YOU'RE
BUSY WITH YOUR JOB. I'M SURE THEY PAY YOU WELL BUT
IT'S A SHAME YOU HAVE TO BE AWAY FROM HOME AND
YOUR FAMILY SO MUCH. HARD TO BELIEVE A YOUNG FEL-
LOW SHOULD HAVE TO WORK SIXTY OR SEVENTY HOURS A
WEEK TO MAKE ENDS MEET. TOO BAD YOU MISSED YOUR
DAUGHTER'S DANCE RECITAL."

HE CONTINUED, "LET ME TELL YOU SOMETHING TOM,
SOMETHING THAT HAS HELPED ME KEEP A GOOD PERSPEC-
TIVE ON MY OWN PRIORITIES."

AND THAT'S WHEN HE BEGAN TO EXPLAIN HIS THEORY
OF A "THOUSAND MARBLES."

"YOU SEE, I SAT DOWN ONE DAY AND DID A LITTLE ARITH-
METIC. THE AVERAGE PERSON LIVES ABOUT SEVENTY-FIVE
YEARS. I KNOW, SOME LIVE MORE AND SOME LIVE LESS,
BUT ON AVERAGE, FOLKS LIVE ABOUT SEVENTY-FIVE YEARS."

"NOW THEN, I MULTIPLIED 75 TIMES 52 AND I CAME UP
WITH 3900 WHICH IS THE NUMBER OF SATURDAYS THAT
THE AVERAGE PERSON HAS IN THEIR ENTIRE LIFETIME. NOW

STICK WITH ME TOM, I'M GETTING TO THE IMPORTANT PART."

"IT TOOK ME UNTIL I WAS FIFTY-FIVE YEARS OLD TO THINK ABOUT ALL THIS IN ANY DETAIL," HE WENT ON, "AND BY THAT TIME I HAD LIVED THROUGH OVER TWENTY-EIGHT HUNDRED SATURDAYS. I GOT TO THINKING THAT IF I LIVED TO BE SEVENTY-FIVE, I ONLY HAD ABOUT A THOUSAND OF THEM LEFT TO ENJOY."

"SO I WENT TO A TOY STORE AND BOUGHT EVERY SINGLE MARBLE THEY HAD. I ENDED UP HAVING TO VISIT THREE TOY STORES TO ROUNDUP 1000 MARBLES. I TOOK THEM HOME AND PUT THEM INSIDE OF A LARGE, CLEAR PLASTIC CONTAINER RIGHT HERE IN THE SHACK NEXT TO MY GEAR. EVERY SATURDAY SINCE THEN, I HAVE TAKEN ONE MARBLE OUT AND THROWN IT AWAY."

"I FOUND THAT BY WATCHING THE MARBLES DIMINISH, I FOCUSED MORE ON THE REALLY IMPORTANT THINGS IN LIFE. THERE IS NOTHING LIKE WATCHING YOUR TIME HERE ON THIS EARTH RUN OUT TO HELP GET YOUR PRIORITIES STRAIGHT."

"NOW LET ME TELL YOU ONE LAST THING BEFORE I SIGN-OFF WITH YOU AND TAKE MY LOVELY WIFE OUT FOR BREAKFAST. THIS MORNING, I TOOK THE VERY LAST MARBLE OUT OF THE CONTAINER. I FIGURE IF I MAKE IT UNTIL NEXT SATURDAY THEN I HAVE BEEN GIVEN A LITTLE EXTRA TIME. AND THE ONE THING WE CAN ALL USE IS A LITTLE MORE TIME."

"IT WAS NICE TO MEET YOU TOM, I HOPE YOU SPEND MORE TIME WITH YOUR FAMILY, AND I HOPE TO MEET YOU AGAIN HERE ON THE BAND. 75 YEAR OLD MAN, THIS IS K9NZQ, CLEAR AND GOING QRT, GOOD MORNING!"

YOU COULD HAVE HEARD A PIN DROP ON THE BAND WHEN THIS FELLOW SIGNED OFF. I GUESS HE GAVE US ALL A LOT TO THINK ABOUT. I HAD PLANNED TO WORK ON THE ANTENNA THAT MORNING, AND THEN I WAS GOING TO MEET

UP WITH A FEW HAMS TO WORK ON THE NEXT CLUB NEWS-
LETTER. INSTEAD, I WENT UPSTAIRS AND WOKE MY WIFE
UP WITH A KISS. "C'MON HONEY, I'M TAKING YOU AND
THE KIDS TO BREAKFAST." "WHAT BROUGHT THIS ON?"
SHE ASKED WITH A SMILE. "OH, NOTHING SPECIAL, IT'S
JUST BEEN A LONG TIME SINCE WE SPENT A SATURDAY TO-
GETHER WITH THE KIDS. HEY, CAN WE STOP AT A TOY
STORE WHILE WE'RE OUT? I NEED TO BUY SOME MARBLES."

CHAPTER 12

How to be a more relaxed person in a freaking-out world

Realizing that I ended up in the Emergency room at the hospital by being out of control and being Type-A personality prone, I was resolute in finding out how not to have that second, or third, and possibly a fatal heart attack again in the future. During my research, I uncovered a case study of Dr. Meyer Friedman, who was working at the Recurrent Coronary Prevention Project in San Francisco's Mt. Zion Hospital (who came up with the original traits of Type-A and Type-B personalities), and who performed a test on 1,013 Type-A personalities and heart attack survivors. He proceeded to place these people into 2 groups. One group of 151 "controls" received the standard care that heart attack survivors would normally receive.

862 patients consented to quit smoking and take either a class on healthy diet or a counseling program, which was developed to change the Type-A personality to that of a Type-B personality. Those that stuck with the counseling program plus the diet program started to notice positive changes in their lives...almost from the outset of the program. They tended to enjoy life more than they had before, their family, friends, and co-workers were happier with them, and they learned to take time every day to stop and relax, to "Stop and smell the Roses" and to just "hang loose."

The most important thing coming out of this revolutionary, and evolutionary program was that the former Type-A's that now had become Type-B's received a special gift the other groups in the test did not receive. The new Type-B's had just half as many of a second, and possibly fatal heart attack over that of the control group.

What can we do NOW to start to migrate from a Type-A to a Type-B personality?

The first thing we all can do is listen to family, friends, and co-workers and stop arguing with them when they all recommend we slow down, smell the flowers, and RELAX. I had to finally realize that the life I am involved with is a work-in-progress. This wondrous journey that we all walk is an unfinished masterpiece. I learned to visualize myself as the painter...savoring each and every brush stroke...but knowing that the masterpiece would never be done.

Stop attempting to do several things at the same time. Not that many people, besides jugglers, can keep three or more balls in the air at the same time... without dropping them. I had to accept that, for the most part, I could do one or two things at one time really well, but if I attempted to have more balls in the air above that number...watch out. One of the greatest tricks I learned, which brought into focus the real priorities in life, was this. I now ask myself which meetings, events, or issues will I care about three to five years from now. I then only do the things that will have meaning years into the future. It's amazing how clear the priority is when you can answer that question.

Forgiveness is very important in learning to be a Type-B person. I had a lot of trouble with that for a lot of years. People would do something that I thought was wrong, and I took it real personally. Heaven forbid that I would forgive them. I used to hold on to anger for years...well beyond even remembering why I was mad. I realized that holding on to anger was only hurting me. So I taught myself how to forgive. I now do it on a daily basis, and it is so freeing to the spirit. If there is anyone in your life that you are holding a grudge against, forgive him or her. You don't have to tell them that you are doing it. They never have to know. Dr. Wayne Dyer, who wrote the book, "Erroneous Zone" says that forgiving is one word, and is two words. One is "forgiving"...and the other is "For Giving." No one has to know you are forgiving and for giving but you. Try it! The rewards are fantastic.

Other things you can do are: Laugh at yourself at least once per day. I am constantly laughing, not only at myself, but also at the world around me. While you are driving, use the time in your car to reflect on the fonder memories of your life. Instead of driving in the far left lane all the time, move over to the far right lane, slow down and enjoy the scenery. If you are in a country that drives on the opposite side of the road than we Americans do...then reverse that procedure.

Learn to be less judgmental. If someone criticizes you, or your actions, don't take it personally. I have learned to support their right to believe the way they choose to believe. Don't get into a verbal fistfight with people...just because you can. No one really wins.

My wife Beth has a placard above her desk that states, "A Rush on your part does not necessitate a rush on mine." In 12 simple words, her placard exemplifies a total cure for being a Type A person.

"Even those of us who are blessed with a large working capacity must realize we cannot exploit ourselves relentlessly...As a human being, I have learned about what a refined instrument the human body and soul is. As Prime Minister, I have learned a lesson about the need to set limits."
                    - Kjell Magne Bondevik -
                    - Prime Minister of Norway -

C H A P T E R 13

More "Control" leads to less stress

We all know people that are as close to living a stress-free life as any human being can get...no matter how crazy the world is that they live in. My wife Beth is one of those people. She is an administrative assistant for a Director at the company she works for in Thousand Oaks, California. Her responsibility is to keep his department running like a finely tuned racecar. Along with those duties, (as if those were not enough to drive the normal person to start drinking heavily), there are 60 to 70 other people that can "pop in" to ask for her assistance on some matter or dire emergency, with no prior warning. At times, the well-intentioned folks expect her to drop the task(s) she is working on and help them out of their crisis...that she does happily and with great pride.

I have observed her in this environment for many years and have never seen her under any sort of real stress. No matter what her circumstances are at the moment, she appears to thrive on the challenge of performing multiple tasks, and all at the same time. It's amazing to watch her work. The more chaos there is, the more efficient and truly calm she becomes. What is her secret? Why do some people have the innate ability to prosper under these types of conditions and others flounder?

I was watching a movie a while ago that illustrates this condition. The movie was "For the Love of the Game" starring Kevin Costner playing the role of a famous baseball figure. I won't go into the play-by-play of the movie. I do recommend you see it. It is a very good and sentimental baseball movie that has a lasting and endearing affect on whomever watches it. Anyway, back to the movie.

Mr. Costner portrays a seasoned baseball pitcher who has been at the top of his game for many years. In one scene...with the stadium filled to capacity, he is standing on the mound...prepared to pitch the ball. The camera pans the audience. The sound is deafening and you wonder how he can concentrate long enough to toss the ball, let alone strike out the batter. The camera pans back to Costner and you hear him say to himself "Filter on"... and the noise from the crowd starts to diminish and finally fades to silence. The camera pans the audience again, this time in total silence. You see the fan's mouths move as if they were yelling, but no sound emanates from them. He is in total "Control" of his surroundings and has trained himself to "filter" out any noises that will distract him from his goal.

Athletes call this "living in the zone." We have all been there at one point in our lives. For me, it's when I used to practice my martial arts at the Aikido dojo I attended. I was concentrating so hard on my "techniques" and focusing on being in total control...and loving it, that I felt zero stress...even though I probably was going to get tossed across the mat in the next second or two.

In my case, I am exactly the opposite of my wife when it comes to how I deal with doing multiple tasks at the same time. I can't! I get really stressed out and end up becoming less effective if put in the same situation as I described Beth thriving in.

So how do I deal with reducing stress brought on by

juggling multiple tasks at once? Looking back at how I was before my heart attack, I was completely out of control of my physical, as well as emotional self, which lead to my ending up in the hospital.

I now have learned that introducing MORE control into your life...not less, as some people tend to believe, REDUCES stress. I have embraced the notion that if you are passionate about your life's work, as my wife is in her career, you enjoy life more, and can thrive in a normally stressful environment as if there were no stress at all.

What if you are not in your ideal job or occupation? How do you "get into the zone" and control your situation? The following tips may be helpful to you; see if one or all fits with your lifestyle.

* Be prepared. If you are an expert at something, you probably are respected, admired, and can rattle off facts about your area of expertise without any stress. Stay up on the latest technology in your field. Keep on the ball, as ball players say.
* Take complete charge of every aspect of your life...not just what interests you.
* "To thine own self be true" - meaning trust in the knowledge you have acquired over the years.
* Listen to your "advisors" but YOU make the final decisions on what is right or wrong. My wife knows "she is right" - it's more than self-confidence, because she listens to her inner voice, and acts on what the voice tells her what needs to be done. Sure, she listens to my feelings, comments and ideas, but, when the pedal needs to hit the metal, she is her own, and best, advisor. I have learned from this and have benefited greatly. Mr. Richard Hatch, actor and motivational speaker,

told me more than once... "All you need to succeed in life...is in you." I agree.

* Don't bite off more than you can chew. Start to control small aspects of your life first, then more, and more, till finally, after you get the hang of it, you have conquered it all. You will be very surprised at how quickly you will accomplish this goal. When you establish a pattern of "Success control", then you end up controlling all aspects of your life, and the by-product is LESS STRESS. Give it a try.

* Do the unspeakable - Ask for help from other people on how you can do better at controlling your own destiny. My greatest advisor is Beth, my wife and best friend. She is also my biggest critic. As she says, "She doesn't lie to, for, or about anyone", and if you don't want to know about how she feels toward a topic, or important matter...then don't ask. She is a "controlling person"...in a positive sense. She says she can only truly be controlling of her own life, and not the lives of others. Again, more control, less stress.

* Control your environment, NOT others. There is an old analogy that will illustrate this concept very clearly. Here it is: Don't try to teach a pig to fly because 1) He is happy being a pig, and 2) To try to control his actions would just make him mad, you'll get stressed out that you can't change him, and ultimately you'll get frustrated.

In reality...the only one you can truly control is you. Learn to do it well, and become an expert at it, and it will change your life.

❤ ❤ ❤

I choose to live
Author unknown

MICHAEL IS THE KIND OF GUY YOU LOVE TO HATE. HE IS ALWAYS IN A GOOD MOOD AND ALWAYS HAS SOMETHING POSITIVE TO SAY. WHEN SOMEONE WOULD ASK HIM HOW HE WAS DOING, HE WOULD REPLY, "IF I WERE ANY BETTER, I WOULD BE TWINS!"

HE WAS A NATURAL MOTIVATOR. IF AN EMPLOYEE WAS HAVING A BAD DAY, MICHAEL WAS THERE TELLING THE EMPLOYEE HOW TO LOOK ON THE POSITIVE SIDE OF THE SITUATION.

SEEING THIS STYLE REALLY MADE ME CURIOUS, SO ONE DAY I WENT UP TO MICHAEL AND ASKED HIM, "I DON'T GET IT! YOU CAN'T BE A POSITIVE PERSON ALL OF THE TIME. HOW DO YOU DO IT?" MICHAEL REPLIED, "EACH MORNING I WAKE UP AND SAY TO MYSELF, MIKE YOU HAVE TWO CHOICES TODAY. YOU CAN CHOOSE TO BE IN A GOOD MOOD OR YOU CAN CHOOSE TO BE IN A BAD MOOD. I CHOOSE TO BE IN A GOOD MOOD.

EACH TIME SOMETHING BAD HAPPENS, I CAN CHOOSE TO BE A VICTIM OR I CAN CHOOSE TO LEARN FROM IT. I CHOOSE TO LEARN FROM IT. EVERY TIME SOMEONE COMES TO ME COMPLAINING, I CAN CHOOSE TO ACCEPT THEIR COMPLAINING OR I CAN POINT OUT THE POSITIVE SIDE OF LIFE. I CHOOSE THE POSITIVE SIDE OF LIFE."

"YEAH, RIGHT, IT'S NOT THAT EASY," I PROTESTED. "YES, IT IS," MICHAEL SAID. "LIFE IS ALL ABOUT CHOICES. WHEN YOU CUT AWAY ALL THE JUNK, EVERY SITUATION IS A CHOICE. YOU CHOOSE HOW YOU REACT TO SITUATIONS. YOU CHOOSE HOW PEOPLE WILL AFFECT YOUR MOOD. YOU CHOOSE TO BE IN A GOOD MOOD OR BAD MOOD. THE BOTTOM LINE: IT'S YOUR CHOICE HOW YOU LIVE LIFE."

I REFLECTED ON WHAT MICHAEL SAID. SOON THEREAF-
TER, I LEFT THE TOWER INDUSTRY TO START MY OWN
BUSINESS. WE LOST TOUCH, BUT I OFTEN THOUGHT ABOUT
HIM THEN I MADE A CHOICE ABOUT LIFE INSTEAD OF RE-
ACTING TO IT.

SEVERAL YEARS LATER, I HEARD THAT MICHAEL WAS
INVOLVED IN A SERIOUS ACCIDENT, FALLING SOME 60 FEET
FROM A COMMUNICATIONS TOWER. AFTER 18 HOURS OF
SURGERY AND WEEKS OF INTENSIVE CARE, MICHAEL WAS
RELEASED FROM THE HOSPITAL WITH RODS PLACED IN HIS
BACK. I SAW MICHAEL ABOUT SIX MONTHS AFTER THE
ACCIDENT.

WHEN I ASKED HIM HOW HE WAS, HE REPLIED. "IF I
WERE ANY BETTER, I'D BE TWINS. WANNA SEE MY SCARS?"
I DECLINED TO SEE HIS WOUNDS, BUT DID ASK HIM WHAT
HAD GONE THROUGH HIS MIND AS THE ACCIDENT TOOK
PLACE. "THE FIRST THING THAT WENT THROUGH MY MIND
WAS THE WELL-BEING OF MY SOON TO BE BORN DAUGH-
TER," MICHAEL REPLIED. "THEN, AS I LAY ON THE
GROUND, I REMEMBERED THAT I HAD TWO CHOICES: I
COULD CHOOSE TO LIVE OR I COULD CHOOSE TO DIE. I
CHOSE TO LIVE."

"WEREN'T YOU SCARED? DID YOU LOSE CONSCIOUS-
NESS?" I ASKED. MICHAEL CONTINUED, "THE PARAMEDICS
WERE GREAT. THEY KEPT TELLING ME I WAS GOING TO BE
FINE. BUT WHEN THEY WHEELED ME INTO THE ER AND I
SAW THE EXPRESSIONS ON THE FACES OF THE DOCTORS AND
NURSES, I GOT REALLY SCARED."

"IN THEIR EYES, I READ 'HE'S A DEAD MAN.' I KNEW I
NEEDED TO TAKE ACTION." "WHAT DID YOU DO?" I ASKED.
"WELL, THERE WAS A BIG BURLY NURSE SHOUTING QUES-
TIONS AT ME," SAID MICHAEL. "SHE ASKED IF I WAS AL-
LERGIC TO ANYTHING."

'YES, I REPLIED." THE DOCTORS AND NURSES STOPPED
WORKING AS THEY WAITED FOR MY REPLY.

I TOOK A DEEP BREATH AND YELLED, "GRAVITY."

OVER THEIR LAUGHTER, I TOLD THEM, "I AM CHOOSING TO LIVE. OPERATE ON ME AS IF I AM ALIVE, NOT DEAD".

MICHAEL LIVED, THANKS TO THE SKILL OF HIS DOCTORS, BUT ALSO BECAUSE OF HIS AMAZING ATTITUDE. I LEARNED FROM HIM THAT EVERY DAY WE HAVE THE CHOICE TO LIVE FULLY.

ATTITUDE, AFTER ALL, IS EVERYTHING. YOU HAVE TWO CHOICES NOW:

1. CHOOSE TO BE IN A GOOD MOOD

2. CHOOSE TO BE IN A BAD MOOD

I HOPE YOU WILL CHOOSE #1. I AM.

CHAPTER 14

Lessons from Fish and Geese

How many times have you heard..."Don't rock the boat" or "Go with the flow" or "Why do you always go against the grain?" Hundreds, I would imagine, but did you really stop to examine what those sayings mean to you and how you deal with life?

I know that the very reason that I ended up in the hospital with a heart attack at a very early age is that I didn't heed that advice. I have been accused of being a bear in a china cabinet. My reputation was one of being inflexible and always doing things my way...even though...as I look back, I was being very stubborn. I thought I had all the answers and knew everything. If I had opened my eyes a little, I would have seen that there were many other ways for me to accomplish my goals if I would have learned to "swim with the fish AND not against the current - but control the flow of the river."

What about that last part of the phase...but control the flow of the river. What do I mean? Lets take the scenario of swimming with the current for a moment. Let's say you did just that... swam with the flow. Wouldn't you get a lot further along down the river than if you were constantly fighting your way upstream? Sure you would.

The problem is that the stream may be going in a direction that is diametrically opposite to the way you want to go. You are going fast, with little stress, but may still miss your mark, ending up further down the river in the wrong direction. So what to do?

The answer is this: Not only swim down the river, but also take over AND control the flow of the river in the direction YOU want the stream to go. If that river doesn't go in the direction you want to go, then find one that does. There are lots of streams and rivers in life that go in all directions. The trick is to find one that works for you...and not the other way around. By finding the right river going in the direction you want to go, you get twice as far, with little or no stress on your part.

But how do you accomplish this? What techniques do you use to swim with the fish AND control the flow of the river? I have included a number of "laws" that might help you "Swim with the fish AND not against the current-but control the flow."

   * There is a universal law that states that the more you flow "with the river" the more people will help you get to where you want to go. People love to help those who know where they are going. We all like winners, optimists, and doers. People like to help and be charitable. Let them. People help those who help themselves.
   * Become singularly focused on your goal. I have found that there are a lot of people who want to stand in your way of success. Don't let the Anti-success mongers get in the way of your dreams.
   * Ask for help and get advice from other people that have successfully arrived and accomplished their goal. This accomplishes two things. 1) It allows you to cut out a whole bunch of lost time trying to figure it out for yourself, and 2) introduces you to someone who can push you along

in the direction you are going. It's kind of like when we were young kids and our parents stood behind us while we sat on the swing in the park. We tried our best to get as much speed and ultimately as high as we could by kicking our legs up in the air. But only when we got a push from behind in the direction that we wanted to go did we get the height we desired. The result was we reached for the stars, and accomplished our goal. Again, ask for help. You will lower you stress level, possibly meet someone new that can help you, and accomplish your goal faster than you ever dreamed possible. I found this illustration on the Internet. LESSONS FROM GEESE" was originally written based on the work of Milton Olson.

"Lessons from Geese"

Fact 1:   As each bird flaps its wings, it creates 'uplift' for the bird following. By flying in a 'V' formation, the whole flock adds 71% greater flying range than if the bird flew alone.

Lesson 1:   People who share a common direction and sense of community can get where they are going quicker and easier because they are traveling on the thrust of one another.

Fact 2:   Whenever a goose falls out of formation, it suddenly feels the draft and resistance of trying to fly alone, and quickly gets back into formation to take advantage of the 'lifting power' of the bird immediately in front.

Lesson 2:   If we have as much sense as a goose we will stay in formation with those who are headed where we want to go (and be willing to accept their help, as well as give ours to the others).

Fact 3:   When the lead goose gets tired, it rotates back into formation and another goose flies at the point position.

Lesson3:   It pays to take turns doing the hard tasks, and sharing leadership with people; as with geese, we are interdependent on each other's skills, capabilities, and unique arrangements of gifts, talents, or resources.

Fact 4:   The geese honk information from behind to encourage those up front to keep up their speed.

Lesson 4:   We need to make sure our honking from behind is encouraging and not something else.

Fact 5:   When a goose gets sick or wounded or shot down, two geese drop out of the formation and follow it down to help and protect it. They stay with it until it is able to fly again or dies. Then they launch out on their own, with another formation, or catch up with the flock.

Lesson 5:   If we have as much sense (and heart) as geese, we too will stand by each other in difficult times as well as when we are strong.

Over the years, I have learned that I can go much farther in life, with less stress, if I surround myself with like-minded, encouraging, and loving people. I have also discovered that If I put their needs ahead of my own, they tend to do the same, and we both benefit. Besides, it's a lot more fun to be going places together, than by yourself.

I am including this story... for one, it's very touching and two, it stresses the point that we should always follow our dreams... no matter how old we get.

♥   ♥   ♥

"Rose"
Author unknown

"THE FIRST DAY OF SCHOOL OUR PROFESSOR INTRODUCED HIMSELF AND CHALLENGED US TO GET TO KNOW SOMEONE WE DIDN'T ALREADY KNOW. I STOOD UP TO LOOK AROUND WHEN A GENTLE HAND TOUCHED MY SHOULDER.

I TURNED AROUND TO FIND A WRINKLED, LITTLE OLD LADY BEAMING UP AT ME WITH A SMILE THAT LIT UP HER ENTIRE BEING. SHE SAID, "HI HANDSOME. MY NAME IS ROSE. I'M EIGHTY-SEVEN YEARS OLD."

"CAN I GIVE YOU A HUG?" I LAUGHED AND ENTHUSIAS-TICALLY RESPONDED, "OF COURSE YOU MAY!" AND SHE GAVE ME A GIANT SQUEEZE.

"WHY ARE YOU IN COLLEGE AT SUCH A YOUNG, INNO-CENT AGE?" I ASKED. SHE JOKINGLY REPLIED, "I'M HERE TO MEET A RICH HUSBAND, GET MARRIED, HAVE A COUPLE OF CHILDREN, AND THEN RETIRE AND TRAVEL."

"NO SERIOUSLY," I ASKED. I WAS CURIOUS WHAT MAY HAVE MOTIVATED HER TO BE TAKING ON THIS CHALLENGE AT HER AGE. "I ALWAYS DREAMED OF HAVING A COLLEGE EDUCATION AND NOW I'M GETTING ONE!" SHE TOLD ME. AFTER CLASS WE WALKED TO THE STUDENT UNION BUILD-ING AND SHARED A CHOCOLATE MILKSHAKE.

WE BECAME INSTANT FRIENDS. EVERY DAY FOR THE NEXT THREE MONTHS WE WOULD LEAVE CLASS TOGETHER AND TALK NONSTOP. I WAS ALWAYS MESMERIZED LISTENING TO THIS "TIME MACHINE" AS SHE SHARED HER WISDOM AND EXPERIENCE WITH ME.

OVER THE COURSE OF THE YEAR, ROSE BECAME A CAMPUS ICON AND SHE EASILY MADE FRIENDS WHEREVER SHE WENT. SHE LOVED TO DRESS UP AND SHE REVELED IN THE ATTENTION BESTOWED UPON HER FROM THE OTHER STUDENTS. SHE WAS LIVING IT UP.

AT THE END OF THE SEMESTER WE INVITED ROSE TO SPEAK AT OUR FOOTBALL BANQUET. I'LL NEVER FORGET WHAT SHE TAUGHT US. SHE WAS INTRODUCED AND STEPPED UP TO THE PODIUM. AS SHE BEGAN TO DELIVER HER PREPARED SPEECH, SHE DROPPED HER THREE BY FIVE CARDS ON THE FLOOR. FRUSTRATED AND A LITTLE EMBARRASSED SHE LEANED INTO THE MICROPHONE AND SIMPLY SAID "I'M SORRY I'M SO JITTERY. I GAVE UP BEER FOR LENT AND THIS WHISKEY IS KILLING ME! I'LL NEVER GET MY SPEECH BACK IN ORDER SO LET ME JUST TELL YOU WHAT I KNOW."

AS WE LAUGHED SHE CLEARED HER THROAT AND BEGAN: "WE DO NOT STOP PLAYING BECAUSE WE ARE OLD; WE GROW OLD BECAUSE WE STOP PLAYING. THERE ARE ONLY FOUR SECRETS TO STAYING YOUNG, BEING HAPPY, AND ACHIEVING SUCCESS." "YOU HAVE TO LAUGH AND FIND HUMOR EVERYDAY." "YOU'VE GOT TO HAVE A DREAM. WHEN YOU LOSE YOUR DREAMS, YOU DIE. WE HAVE SO MANY PEOPLE WALKING AROUND WHO ARE DEAD AND DON'T EVEN KNOW IT!" "THERE IS A HUGE DIFFERENCE BETWEEN GROWING OLDER AND GROWING UP. IF YOU ARE NINETEEN YEARS OLD AND LIE IN BED FOR ONE FULL YEAR AND DON'T DO ONE PRODUCTIVE THING, YOU WILL TURN TWENTY YEARS OLD. IF I AM EIGHTY-SEVEN YEARS OLD AND STAY IN BED FOR A YEAR AND NEVER DO ANYTHING I WILL TURN EIGHTY-EIGHT. ANYBODY CAN GROW OLDER. THAT DOESN'T TAKE ANY TALENT OR ABILITY. THE IDEA IS TO GROW UP BY ALWAYS FINDING THE OPPORTUNITY IN CHANGE."

"HAVE NO REGRETS. THE ELDERLY USUALLY DON'T HAVE REGRETS FOR WHAT WE DID, BUT RATHER FOR THINGS WE DID NOT DO. THE ONLY PEOPLE WHO FEAR DEATH ARE THOSE WITH REGRETS."

SHE CONCLUDED HER SPEECH BY COURAGEOUSLY SING-
ING "THE ROSE." SHE CHALLENGED EACH OF US TO STUDY
THE LYRICS AND LIVE THEM OUT IN OUR DAILY LIVES.

AT YEAR'S END ROSE FINISHED THE COLLEGE DEGREE
SHE HAD BEGUN ALL THOSE YEARS AGO.

ONE WEEK AFTER GRADUATION ROSE DIED PEACEFULLY
IN HER SLEEP.

OVER TWO THOUSAND COLLEGE STUDENTS ATTENDED
HER FUNERAL IN TRIBUTE TO THE WONDERFUL WOMAN
WHO TAUGHT BY EXAMPLE THAT IT'S NEVER TOO LATE TO
BE ALL YOU CAN POSSIBLY BE. IF YOU READ THIS, PLEASE
SEND THIS PEACEFUL WORD OF ADVICE TO YOUR FRIENDS
AND FAMILY, THEY'LL REALLY ENJOY IT! WE SEND THESE
WORDS IN LOVING MEMORY OF ROSE. REMEMBER, GROW-
ING OLDER IS MANDATORY, GROWING UP IS
OPTIONAL.

HOPE YOUR LIFE HAS A LITTLE ROSE IN IT, ALSO.

15

Attitude IS everything
Not just a point of view

Before I get into the meat of this chapter, I want to interject a small article called "Attitude" by Charles Swindol. I could write volumes on the strength of this paragraph and Charles' concept of attitude and how to deal with life's issues. So here it is in its entirety.

"The longer I live, the more I realize the impact of attitude on life. Attitude to me is more important than facts. It is more important than the past, than education, than money, than circumstances, than failure, than successes, than what other people think or say or do. It is more important than appearance, giftedness or skill. It will make or break a company... a church...a home. The remarkable thing is we have a choice every day regarding the Attitude we will embrace for that day. We cannot change our past. We cannot change the fact that people will act in a certain way. We cannot change the inevitable. The only thing we can do is play on the one string we have, and that is our Attitude. I am convinced that life is 10% what happens to me and 90% how I react to it."

And so it is with you. We are in charge of our Attitude. Most people I talk to about this topic have a very strong sense about what the statement is all about in reference to how we deal with the failures in our lives. It's all about our attitude toward these failures, or setbacks, and how we deal with these setbacks that either holds us back, or motivates us to be the best we can be, reaching for the stars, and accomplishing anything our hearts and minds can conceive.

When I talked about this to a co-worker the other day, he stated that failure is "The end." Once you give it your all, and fail anyway, the game is over, finished, end-of-story. His feelings about this are not at all an isolated case. I cannot tell you how many people have been brought up to think this way about failure, from when they were children and now have carried this into adulthood.

Can you even imagine if some of the greatest minds throughout history had adopted this point of view? How about all the painters, writers, musicians, sculptors, inventors, and thinkers that we have heard about our entire lives? How about Honest Abe Lincoln, Thomas Edison, Socrates, and Einstein, to name just a few? In Edison's case, he tried over 10,000 times to test different filaments in the light bulbs he was inventing before he found the right combination.   If he had given up, became really stressed out, and not gone any further, you might be reading this book using a candle as a light source. Honest Abe tried and tried again to run for President of the United States unsuccessfully until he finally succeeded. Just imagine if he, too, had given up. He would have stayed in obscurity, and the world would have been deprived of one its greatest statesmen.

Success in anything you do has to do with having a positive Attitude. Plain and simple, attitude is the engine that gets you going in the right direction and for the right reason. Think about it this way; if you think about failure in relation to a timeline where you set a goal and fail at it after only one attempt...and you don't get up and try again...that's the END. THE FINISH...PERIOD. You have displayed the attitude that failure is the norm.

Your self-talk goes something like this "well, I tried, and failed. I guess it just wasn't meant to be." Think of all the times we tried something just once, and gave up and remember how much STRESS came out of that sad day.

But now let's take that same timeline and goal used in the first example. This time, when you stumble and fall, you pick yourself up, brush yourself off, and go at the goal again and again until you succeed. Each time you get up and go after it again, you are saying I can do it, am willing to try again and again, until I succeed. YOUR attitude is 180 degrees opposite from the first example. You look at this problem, and life, as a set of steps to your goals. If you know full well that you will continue until you succeed, falling down is just a small bump in the road. Failure is just a small inconvenient event on your journey.

The next time you have a goal in mind, and stumble a little bit while reaching for that goal, just get back up, brush yourself off and try it again, and again until you accomplish what you set out to do. You will be amazed at how little stress (if any) creeps into your life, if you adopt this new approach to failure - as only an event on your way to success.

As a side note; you may notice that you may not be falling down as much as you THINK, after you adopt this new way of approaching failure.

ACHIEVING 100% IN LIFE
Author Uknown

WE HAVE ALL BEEN TO THOSE MEETINGS WHERE SOMEONE WANTS YOU TO ACHIEVE *100%*

HERE'S HOW YOU CAN ACHIEVE 100%. FIRST OF ALL, HERE'S A LITTLE MATH THAT MIGHT PROVE HELPFUL IN THE FUTURE: HOW DOES ONE ACHIEVE 100% IN LIFE?

BEGIN BY NOTING THE FOLLOWING:

IF:

A = 1	J = 10	S = 19
B = 2	K = 11	T = 20
C = 3	L = 12	U = 21
D = 4	M = 13	V = 22
E = 5	N = 14	W = 23
F = 6	O = 15	X = 24
G = 7	P = 16	Y = 25
H = 8	Q = 17	Z = 26
I = 9	R = 18	

THEN,

H A R D W O R K

$8 + 1 + 18 + 4 + 23 + 15 + 18 + 11 =$ ONLY 98%

SIMILARLY,

K N O W L E D G E

$11 + 14 + 15 + 23 + 12 + 5 + 4 + 7 + 5 =$ ONLY 96%

BUT INTERESTING (AND AS YOU'D EXPECT),

A T T I T U D E

$1 + 20 + 20 + 9 + 20 + 21 + 4 + 5 = 100\%$

THIS IS HOW YOU ACHIEVE 100% IN LIFE

♥   ♥   ♥

THE WINDOW
Author unknown

A GREAT NOTE FOR ALL TO READ. IT WILL TAKE JUST
30 SECOND TO READ THIS AND CHANGE YOUR THINKING.
TWO MEN, BOTH SERIOUSLY ILL, OCCUPIED THE SAME
HOSPITAL ROOM. ONE MAN WAS ALLOWED TO SIT UP IN
HIS BED FOR AN HOUR EACH AFTERNOON TO HELP DRAIN
THE FLUID FROM HIS LUNGS. HIS BED WAS NEXT TO THE
ROOM'S ONLY WINDOW. THE OTHER MAN HAD TO SPEND
ALL HIS TIME FLAT ON HIS BACK. THE MEN TALKED FOR
HOURS ON END. THEY SPOKE OF THEIR WIVES AND FAMI-
LIES, THEIR HOMES, THEIR JOBS, THEIR INVOLVEMENT IN
THE MILITARY SERVICE, WHERE THEY HAD BEEN ON VACA-
TION.

EVERY AFTERNOON WHEN THE MAN IN THE BED BY THE
WINDOW COULD SIT UP, HE WOULD PASS THE TIME BY DE-
SCRIBING TO HIS ROOMMATE ALL THE THINGS HE COULD
SEE OUTSIDE THE WINDOW. THE MAN IN THE OTHER BED
BEGAN TO LIVE, FOR THOSE ONE-HOUR PERIODS WHERE HIS
WORLD WOULD BE BROADENED AND ENLIVENED BY ALL
THE ACTIVITY AND COLOR OF THE WORLD OUTSIDE. THE
WINDOW OVERLOOKED A PARK WITH A LOVELY LAKE. DUCKS
AND SWANS PLAYED ON THE WATER WHILE CHILDREN SAILED
THEIR MODEL BOATS. YOUNG LOVERS WALKED ARM IN
ARM AMIDST FLOWERS OF EVERY COLOR OF THE RAINBOW.
GRAND OLD TREES GRACED THE LANDSCAPE, AND A FINE
VIEW OF THE CITY SKYLINE COULD BE SEEN IN THE DIS-
TANCE. AS THE MAN BY THE WINDOW DESCRIBED ALL
THIS IN EXQUISITE DETAIL, THE MAN ON THE OTHER SIDE
OF THE ROOM WOULD CLOSE HIS EYES AND IMAGINE THE
PICTURESQUE SCENE.

ONE WARM AFTERNOON THE MAN BY THE WINDOW DE-
SCRIBED A PARADE PASSING BY. ALTHOUGH THE OTHER MAN

COULDN'T HEAR THE BAND - HE COULD SEE IT. IN HIS MIND'S EYE AS THE GENTLEMAN BY THE WINDOW PORTRAYED IT WITH DESCRIPTIVE WORDS.

DAYS AND WEEKS PASSED. ONE MORNING THE DAY NURSE ARRIVED TO BRING WATER FOR THEIR BATHS ONLY TO FIND THE LIFELESS BODY OF THE MAN BY THE WINDOW, WHO HAD DIED PEACE-FULLY IN HIS SLEEP. SHE WAS SADDENED AND CALLED THE HOSPITAL ATTENDANTS TO TAKE THE BODY AWAY. AS SOON AS IT SEEMED APPROPRIATE, THE OTHER MAN ASKED IF HE COULD BE MOVED NEXT TO THE WINDOW. THE NURSE WAS HAPPY TO MAKE THE SWITCH, AND AFTER MAKING SURE HE WAS COMFORTABLE, SHE LEFT HIM ALONE. SLOWLY PAINFULLY, HE PROPPED HIMSELF UP ON ONE ELBOW TO TAKE HIS FIRST LOOK AT THE WORLD OUTSIDE. FINALLY, HE WOULD HAVE THE JOY OF SEEING IT FOR HIMSELF. HE STRAINED TO SLOWLY TURN TO LOOK OUT THE WINDOW BESIDE THE BED. IT FACED A BLANK WALL.

THE MAN ASKED THE NURSE WHAT COULD HAVE COMPELLED HIS DECEASED ROOMMATE WHO HAD DESCRIBED SUCH WONDERFUL THINGS OUTSIDE THIS WINDOW. THE NURSE RESPONDED THAT THE MAN WAS BLIND AND COULD NOT EVEN SEE THE WALL. SHE SAID, "PERHAPS HE JUST WANTED TO ENCOURAGE YOU."

EPILOGUE: THERE IS TREMENDOUS HAPPINESS IN MAKING OTHERS HAPPY, DESPITE OUR OWN SITUATIONS. SHARED GRIEF IS HALF THE SORROW, BUT HAPPINESS WHEN SHARED, IS DOUBLED. IF YOU WANT TO FEEL RICH, JUST COUNT ALL THE THINGS YOU HAVE THAT MONEY CAN'T BUY. "TODAY IS A GIFT, THAT'S WHY IT IS CALLED THE PRESENT."

CHAPTER 16

CHAPTER 16

Dealing with Priorities

My wife and I decided to do something really spec
tacular for the new Millennium to celebrate the turn
of the century. After exhaustive research about what
would be fun and exciting, we opted to take a cruise
through the South Pacific and place ourselves in the part
of the world that became the year 2000 first. One of the
stops on our agenda was to tour a mountain lake area
called Cradle Lake in New Zealand. The tour guide was
a bearded chap with a leather hat and a look right out of
the movie "Crocodile Dundee." He and I got to into a
conversation about how relaxed everyone was that lived
in New Zealand, and how different that was from my
perception of how Americans generally are. He indicated that it "all had to do with pri-or-ities - mate."

Probing further, he gave me his philosophy, and sage
advice that he had learned over the years. Here it is in a
nutshell. "If you can accomplish a goal the first
day...great. If not, do it on the second day. If you can't
get it done by the end of the 2nd day, it isn't worth doing
anyway, mate, so just forget about it altogether...cause it
wasn't worth doing anyhow."

There is a lot to be said for his way of thinking. We
tend to take on more and more "stuff" in our lives that
we feel needs to be done... without really examining how

important the goals are and how NOT doing them will impact our lives. My feeling is that when I start to pile more and more goals on top of already existing goals, I get really stressed out and like the juggler with too many balls in the air at one time, I tend to drop some.

Over the years I have devised a very simple, but effective, way to not only set goals but also accomplish them... and have fun and feel like I got something done when the end of the day came. Before I give you my secret to great goal settings, I want to state this disclaimer. There are a lot of wonderful time management systems on the market today to keep track of your goals, contact lists, and to prioritize dealing with people, places and things. I am not advocating tossing them out and using my system cold turkey. If you choose to try out the system I propose, use it to work on fun projects and use your existing management system for work. When you get the hang of the system, you might choose to use it for work. So here it goes.

Get yourself a package of three by five cards from the stationary store. Then think of a number between 3 and 5 that you feel VERY comfortable with. My number is 3. This number is how many goals you honestly think you accomplish without getting stressed out. If you think that even five is a number that is too small for you type "A" personalities, remember why you are reading this book. Remember you had a heart attack and it was probably due to you being too goal hungry.

Now that you have the three by five cards, open up the package and on the first card, write down the goal that you want to accomplish. What's important here is to be VERY clear on the end result. Don't say you want to be rich, but rather state the goal as "I will have $1,000,000 in the bank when I reach my 49th birthday." On the back of the card outline HOW you THINK you will accomplish this. Do this for all three of your most important goals you have AT THIS MOMENT. Read the card (front and back) three times immediately after you create the card. It is proven that habits are formulated by repeating the actions a number of times until it becomes entrenched into our subconscious mind. I also want you to read each goal card three times - three times per day. This will permanently cement the goal into your mind.

After I have created these three goals, I place them in my shirt pocket (assuming you have a shirt pocket). I focus on these goals, and ONLY these goals. Here is the fun part. I get a small container and place it in a obvious place at work (or home).

When I complete the goal, I place the completed card in the container. I then create another goal card and place the new one in my shirt pocket to replace the one I have completed. (Voila!) Using this system, I have cut down the stress of goal setting over that of using more complicated systems...and kept it SIMPLE. It is amazing how many goals I have in my goal container at the end of the day, week, or month. The secret to this simple system is to have fun with it but be specific with what you strive for.

The reality is that the only true priority in our lives is to get up, eat enough food to get by, be loved, give love, have fun, and be happy. All the other priorities in life are "add-ons."

❤ ❤ ❤

Another "Take a Look At Yourself" Story...
Author unknown

ABOUT TEN YEARS AGO, A YOUNG AND VERY SUCCESS-FUL EXECUTIVE NAMED JOSH WAS TRAVELING DOWN A CHICAGO NEIGHBORHOOD STREET. HE WAS GOING A BIT TOO FAST IN HIS SLEEK, BLACK, 12 CYLINDER JAGUAR XKE, WHICH WAS ONLY TWO MONTHS OLD.

HE WAS WATCHING FOR KIDS DARTING OUT FROM BE-TWEEN PARKED CARS AND SLOWED DOWN WHEN HE THOUGHT HE SAW SOMETHING. AS HIS CAR PASSED, NO CHILD DARTED OUT, BUT A BRICK SAILED OUT AND-WHUMP!-IT SMASHED INTO THE JAG'S SHINY BLACK SIDE DOOR!

SCREECH...!!!! BRAKES SLAMMED! GEARS GROUND INTO REVERSE, AND TIRES MADLY SPUN THE JAGUAR BACK TO THE SPOT FROM WHERE THE BRICK HAD BEEN THROWN.

JOSH JUMPED OUT OF THE CAR, GRABBED THE KID AND PUSHED HIM UP AGAINST A PARKED CAR. HE SHOUTED AT THE KID, "WHAT WAS THAT ALL ABOUT AND WHO ARE YOU? JUST WHAT THE HECK ARE YOU DOING?!" BUILDING UP A HEAD OF STEAM, HE WENT ON. "THAT'S MY NEW JAG, THAT BRICK YOU THREW IS GONNA COST YOU A LOT OF MONEY. WHY DID YOU THROW IT?"

"PLEASE, MISTER, PLEASE ... I'M SORRY! I DIDN'T KNOW WHAT ELSE TO DO!" PLEADED THE YOUNGSTER. "I THREW THE BRICK BECAUSE NO ONE ELSE WOULD STOP!" TEARS WERE DRIPPING DOWN THE BOY'S CHIN AS HE POINTED AROUND THE PARKED CAR. "IT'S MY BROTHER, MISTER," HE SAID. "HE ROLLED OFF THE CURB AND FELL OUT OF HIS WHEELCHAIR AND I CAN'T LIFT HIM UP." SOBBING, THE BOY ASKED THE EXECUTIVE, "WOULD YOU PLEASE HELP ME GET HIM BACK INTO HIS WHEELCHAIR? HE'S HURT AND HE'S TOO HEAVY FOR ME."

MOVED BEYOND WORDS, THE YOUNG EXECUTIVE TRIED DESPERATELY TO SWALLOW THE RAPIDLY SWELLING LUMP IN HIS THROAT. STRAINING, HE LIFTED THE YOUNG MAN BACK INTO THE WHEELCHAIR AND TOOK OUT HIS HAND-KERCHIEF AND WIPED THE SCRAPES AND CUTS, CHECKING TO SEE THAT EVERYTHING WAS GOING TO BE OK. HE THEN WATCHED THE YOUNGER BROTHER PUSH HIM DOWN THE SIDEWALK TOWARD THEIR HOME.

IT WAS A LONG WALK BACK TO THE SLEEK, BLACK, SHIN-ING, 12 CYLINDER JAGUAR XKE-A LONG AND SLOW WALK. JOSH NEVER DID FIX THE SIDE DOOR OF HIS JAGUAR. HE KEPT THE DENT TO REMIND HIM NOT TO GO THROUGH LIFE SO FAST THAT SOMEONE HAS TO THROW A BRICK AT HIM TO GET HIS ATTENTION...

CHAPTER 17

Compete with yourself - Not with others

Have you ever watched the Special Olympics on TV or in person? If you haven't, I encourage you to the next time it airs on television, or comes into town. There are all these wonderful and very special people competing in an assortment of athletic events... and having the time of their lives doing it. They all appear to be like the "Three Musketeers" - one for all and all for one. The kids could care less about winning the races they are entered into by beating the other runners to the finish line. I watched one event where one little fellow fell down during the race and low and behold... all the other runners STOPPED, went back, picked up the competitor, and they all crossed the finish line together, arm-in-arm, singing all the while. I could hardly hold back my tears.

Each child was not concerned in the least about beating out the other runners and winning the race. Each one was only competing with himself or herself. All they wanted to do was be the best they could be and do the best they could do with the talent they possessed. Much more important than winning was their concern for another human being in trouble. What a lesson we could all learn by emulating their behavior on and off the field.

When I was in high school, I was on the Cross Country Track team. Every week we had a competition between our school, and other schools in the San Fernando Valley, just north of Los Angeles, California. My coach was a wonderful mentor to all of us, but particularly encouraging to a tall, lanky, first year high school student. Me. He would preach to us continually of the virtue of "only competing with yourself because no one else matters." I was probably cocky enough to think "yeah right", as if most teenagers would accept that notion by anyone of his generation.

We were entered into a race with a team of superior athletic ability, and we knew we were going to get pounced, and beaten to a pulp (athletically speaking that is). My race, or "heat" was against three High School senior athletes from the other school, who eventually came in first, second, and third in the foot race. I was devastated. I gave it my best effort...my all, but was clobbered anyway.

I remember going to the coach with my fourth place ribbon in hand, embarrassed that I had performed so poorly. His response was one of total surprise. He said how proud he was that I won the race. I said I came in fourth place, so how could I be called a winner? He asked me if I gave it my ALL and I said I did. He then asked me if there was anything else I could have done to change the outcome of the race. I said "besides having the kids assassinated before they ran," I said I did everything I could to run the race and if I had to do it over again, I would have run it the same way. The coach said I was then the winner because you were only competing with yourself.

How many times in our lives do we see and know other people who are better, or richer, or taller, or shorter, than we are and dream we could be just like them?

There will always be someone with more "stuff" than you or I have. Someone who is richer, taller, shorter, thinner, or wiser than we think we are. Accept it. This is so important that I want to repeat it again. There will always be someone with more "stuff" than you or I have. Who is richer, taller, shorter, thinner, or wiser than we think we are. Accept it.

I am not advocating giving up and accepting the lot in life that you have been dealt. That is not at all the message that I am conveying here. I am saying that it's okay to strive for a better walk in life, as long as you do it for you and not because of your parents, your spouse, your family, or for what your friends want, or expect, you to be. Accept who you are today, and strive to be better tomorrow...and do it for the one and only person who is the most important person in your life...and that person is ONLY you.

Remember the Special Olympic kids in the beginning of this story? Learn the lessons that those very special kids who participated in the Special Olympics have learned, and embraced. Lower your stress level by doing the best you can do, and know that in your heart you are a winner. Always have been and always will be.

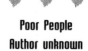

Poor People
Author unknown

ONE DAY A FATHER OF A VERY WEALTHY FAMILY TOOK HIS SON ON A TRIP TO THE COUNTRY WITH THE FIRM PURPOSE OF SHOWING HIS SON HOW POOR PEOPLE CAN BE. THEY SPENT A COUPLE OF DAYS AND NIGHTS ON THE FARM OF WHAT WOULD BE CONSIDERED A VERY POOR FAMILY.

ON THEIR RETURN FROM THEIR TRIP, THE FATHER ASKED HIS SON, "HOW WAS THE TRIP?" "IT WAS GREAT, DAD." "DID YOU SEE HOW POOR PEOPLE CAN BE?" THE FATHER

ASKED. "OH YEAH" SAID THE SON. "SO WHAT DID YOU LEARN FROM THE TRIP?" ASKED THE FATHER.

THE SON ANSWERED, "I SAW THAT WE HAVE ONE DOG AND THEY HAD FOUR." "WE HAVE A POOL THAT REACHES TO THE MIDDLE OF OUR GARDEN AND THEY HAVE A CREEK THAT HAS NO END." "WE HAVE IMPORTED LANTERNS IN OUR GARDEN AND THEY HAVE THE STARS AT NIGHT." "OUR PATIO REACHES TO THE FRONT YARD AND THEY HAVE THE WHOLE HORIZON."

"WE HAVE A SMALL PIECE OF LAND TO LIVE ON AND THEY HAVE FIELDS THAT GO BEYOND OUR SIGHT." "WE HAVE SERVANTS WHO SERVE US, BUT THEY SERVE OTHERS." "WE BUY OUR FOOD, BUT THEY GROW THEIRS."

"WE HAVE WALLS AROUND OUR PROPERTY TO PROTECT US, THEY HAVE FRIENDS TO PROTECT THEM." WITH THIS THE BOY'S FATHER WAS SPEECHLESS.

THEN HIS SON ADDED, "THANKS DAD FOR SHOWING ME HOW POOR WE ARE." TOO MANY TIMES WE FORGET WHAT WE HAVE AND CONCENTRATE ON WHAT WE DON'T HAVE. WHAT IS ONE PERSON'S WORTHLESS OBJECT IS ANOTHER'S PRIZE POSSESSION. IT IS ALL BASED ON ONE'S PERSPECTIVE. MAKES YOU WONDER WHAT WOULD HAPPEN IF WE ALL GAVE THANKS TO GOD FOR ALL THE BOUNTY WE HAVE BEEN PROVIDED BY HIM, INSTEAD OF WORRYING ABOUT WANTING MORE.

C H A P T E R 18

One dollar for a dollar problem
$100 for a $100 dollar problem©

Don't make a mountain out of a molehill, and other such analogies like these have been around for decades and we all have heard them... starting at an early age...from our parents to our schoolteachers and managers at our places of employment. No matter how it is stated, the underlying theme is the same. We humans tend to make far more of a situation than the situation really warrants.

I remember, as a young man, that my father traveled a lot for his business. Being a rambunctious lad, I probably got in trouble more than I now remember. There was one time - when just before Dad went on one of those business trips, he caught me doing something terribly wrong but didn't have time to discipline me before he left. So he did what I would imagine fathers around the world do and said "I will deal with this when I get home" and proceeded to leave the house for parts unknown.

Since Mom didn't hear the conversation, she had no idea what happened and worse than that, couldn't figure out what the punishment would be when he came back. By the time dad had returned from his travels about three weeks later I had worried myself to death, getting no sleep, and fretting the entire time about how my life was to change due to the severe repercussions for my misbehaving. Then dad stepped through the door.

If I remember correctly, he grounded me for a day and never brought up the subject again. Being a father as I am now, I now believe that he knew exactly what he was doing when he left the house that day. He knew I would sweat and fret about my actions and...that action alone would have been the lesson. I am sure that whatever I did before he left never happened again after he returned.

I have told that story to make a point, and of course the point is that we make mountains out of molehills all the time. This action is the one that adds stress to our lives and if we can learn to see the situation for what it really is, we are then more in-tune to a better outcome.

And what do I mean by "One dollar for a dollar problem-$100 for a $100 problem?" Here is the secret to dealing with those mountains and molehills and controlling the stress in your lives when they are placed in your path.

Think of problems with a value system placed on them. A one-dollar problem would equate to a molehill type of problem, and a $100 dollar problem would be the mountain type of problem. Where we get into trouble is investing $100 dollars of our energy, brainpower, and total self into what is really a one-dollar problem. OR conversely, investing one dollar into a $100 problem. We either take the problem too seriously, or not seriously enough. Either scenario can lead to meltdown and enormous impact to both physical and mental state of being. So, the next time a problem comes up, think of the problem in the context of investing and the return on your investment. Take a dollar bill out of your wallet, and really look at it for a moment. Every time you see a dollar bill on a billboard, TV commercial, or in you wallet, think of it as the greatest tool for dealing with problems. Think of what you are getting for your buck.

❦   ❦   ❦

♥   ♥   ♥

The secret of health for both mind and body is not to mourn for the past, nor to worry about the future, nor to anticipate trouble, but to live the present moment wisely and earnestly.

– Buddha –

CHAPTER 19

CHAPTER 19

Say no, and really mean it
Assertiveness training 101

Have you ever been in a situation where you wanted to be assertive, take a stand for some cause, but at the last minute backed down? I suspect we all have. While standing around the coffee pot, we tell our co-workers how we are going to march right into the boss' office, lean across the mahogany desk, and tell him you want a raise. All your friends support your newfound courage, and egg you on to do what you have bragged about doing. After your "tribe" rants and raves about how right you are...you muster up the fortitude, stroll into your leader's office, to ultimately peter out at the last moment. He had you right where he wanted you, didn't he?

Perhaps this scenario hasn't happened to you exactly as I have described it, but, face it, we all have had moments where being assertive would have pushed our career, and/ or our family relationship up to a higher, more meaningful level.

Take my advice, and learn to be more assertive. Not being assertive will allow people to tromp all over you unnecessarily. Learn to say "No" when you don't want to do something you feel is unreasonable and goes against your inner feeling of what is right or wrong. Standing up for your belief systems, and being assertive allows you to respect yourself and others. Have you noticed that assertive people have tons of self-confidence? Even when they make mistakes, or fall down, they have enough self-confidence to pick themselves back up, and go on. They even take responsibility for their actions. Assertive people may be disappointed with their failures, but their confidence level remains high through thick and thin.

I have observed that people who have mastered the art of assertiveness are very much in touch with their emotions and have learned to release any negative emotional baggage, while keeping stress in check.

Let's re-examine the situation I described above with perhaps a different outcome. For this example, we make the assumption you have been through a course entitled "Assertiveness Training 101." The first thing I would do is not brag your intentions to the "tribe". Quiet action speaks volumes over being a blowhard. People tend to respect quietly assertive individuals. If you are at the coffee pot, and must say something to the group when asked what your meeting is all about, you might state something like, "he asked for my guidance of subject X, Y, or Z"...and leave it at that. Remember, keeping a secret is all part of the fun.

Instead of marching into the office with both barrels blazing...have a plan, make an appointment, and inform your boss ahead of time what the meeting is all about. You don't like to be surprised, and neither does he, right? Now, keep your appointment, be on time, and act calmly assertive. Tell him what he can expect from the conversation, be matter-of-fact, and by all means, be professional. Being calmly assertive will tell him you are self confident in your actions. He cannot help noticing that

Know your limits... and be PREPARED to live within them
- Brad Henson -

you are a changed person who knows exactly what you want. Inform him you deserve the raise because you are fully qualified, and then you produce hard-core proof to substantiate your claims. In just a few minutes, you have gotten your raise, not by bullying your boss, but by being assertive, self confident, and knowing what you want.

If you are in a situation where someone asks you to do something that you do not want or have the time to do, be assertive, polite and just say "no." In this situation, give the person asking an alternative action to follow. This way, they go away with a good feeling about you, and a possible solution to their problem. Who knows, they may come back to you in the future knowing full well you can't do what they are asking ...but would be willing to assist them with their problem, in the end, solving two problems for the price of one.

The bottom line is this: Until you stand up for yourself, and become more assertive, you will be walked on, have poor self esteem, and put your body under tremendous stress. Allowing this kind of behavior to continually occur over time will release more stressors into the blood stream, lead to increased occurrences of anger, which may then lead to heart disease, or other ailments.

By just saying "No" and meaning it, could help you avoid all of this ...and remember, it really is an art.

Received via email
Michael and Marsha Pearson

I HAD A VERY SPECIAL TEACHER IN SCHOOL YEARS AGO WHOSE HUSBAND UNEXPECTEDLY DIED OF A HEART ATTACK. ABOUT A WEEK AFTER HIS DEATH, SHE SHARED SOME OF HER INSIGHT WITH A CLASSROOM OF STUDENTS.

As the late afternoon sunlight came streaming in through the classroom windows and class was nearly over, she moved a few things aside on the edge of her desk and sat down there.

With a gentle look of reflection on her face, she paused and said, "Before class is over, I would like to share with all of you a thought that is unrelated to class, but which I feel very important. Each of us is put here on earth to learn, share, love, appreciate and give of ourselves. None of us knows when this fantastic experience will end. It can be taken away any moment. Perhaps this is God's way of telling us that we must make the most out of every single day."

Her eyes beginning to tear, she went on, "So I would like you all to make me a promise."

"From now on, on your way to school, or on your way home, find something beautiful to notice. It doesn't have to be something you see, it could be a scent, perhaps of freshly baked bread wafting out of someone's house, or it could be the sound of a breeze slightly rustling the leaves in the trees, or the way the morning light catches one autumn leaf as it falls gently to the ground. Please look for these things, and cherish them." "For, although it may sound trite to some, these things are the 'stuff' of life. The little things we are put here on earth to enjoy. The things we often take for granted. We must make it important to notice them, for at any time, it can all be taken away." The class was completely quiet. We all picked up our books and filed out of the room silently. That afternoon, I noticed more things on my way home from school than I had that whole semester. Every once in a while, I think of that teacher and remember what

AN IMPRESSION SHE MADE ON ALL OF US, AND I TRY TO APPRECIATE ALL OF THOSE THINGS THAT SOMETIMES WE ALL OVERLOOK. TAKE NOTICE OF SOMETHING SPECIAL YOU SEE ON YOUR LUNCH HOUR TODAY. GO BAREFOOT. OR WALK ON THE BEACH AT SUNSET. STOP OFF ON THE WAY HOME TONIGHT TO GET A DOUBLE-DIP ICE CREAM CONE. FOR AS WE GET OLDER, IT IS NOT THE THINGS WE DID THAT WE OFTEN REGRET, BUT THE THINGS WE DIDN'T DO. IF YOU LIKE THIS, PLEASE PASS IT ON TO A FRIEND, IF NOT, JUST DELETE IT. LIFE IS NOT MEASURED BY THE NUMBER OF BREATHS WE TAKE, BUT BY THE MOMENTS THAT TAKE OUR BREATH AWAY.

C H A P T E R 20

Know when to hold em, know when to fold em
Know when to walk away

Know when to walk away! Sometimes we find ourselves staying longer on a project, in a relationship or a situation than we should. The result of this action may be a lessening of impact to the project, a lower return on our investment, words said that can never be taken back (in cases of arguments), a potential loss of revenue, or loss of status within the corporate environment where we work...ultimately adding gobs of stress into our lives. This stress results in hurt feelings, increases costs, reduces profit to our mental well being, and most likely causes higher blood pressure.

Men learn early the concept of cutting their losses if the project doesn't work out. It's called dating. A guy meets a girl, sets up a date, and buys a bushel of flowers to blanket the girl with love and affection. After the initial outlay of hard earned money the girl doesn't like the guy, or the guy doesn't like the girl, he dumps her, cuts his losses and goes on to the next "date", and the cycle repeats itself. Even at an earlier age, both boys and girls vie for the affection of their mom and dad. They learn what techniques work, and which ones don't. As we get older, we take those lessons with us into other relationships, be it work-related or personal encounters. At work, we size up our bosses and co-workers to see how much mileage we can get by using time-tested techniques from our youth.

If you need to assess the status of a project, ask the following questions at numerous steps of the project, determine the point at which you should cut and run, or stay the course to completion.

* Is there anything you could or should have done that would make the outcome happen in your favor?
* Is there anything that someone ELSE could or should have done that would make the outcome turn out the way YOU wanted it to?
* Is there anything you didn't know that affected the way the project turned out...and if you did know that fact, could you have used it to make the project turn out better?

Learn to evaluate the situation for what it really is...not the way you expect or wish it to be. We always get into trouble when our expectation outweighs reality.

When I come up against an issue that needs a go/no go evaluation, I first ask what is the worst thing that can happen if this project is canceled? Once I accept the worst-case scenario, then the outcome doesn't seem so bad. I then ask the three questions above weighing each one from 1 to 5, where 1 has the least impact to the outcome, and 5 being the heaviest impact and a project stopper.

At times, the go/no go test takes hours, and other times, (depending on the simplicity and/or complexity of the problem) the process takes just seconds. Either way, just the very act of taking action lessens the stressors, brings into focus the real issues that need to be addressed, or not addressed, and a clear view from which you can make a sound and rational decision.

As Kenny Rogers sang "Know when to hold em, know when to fold em...and know when to walk away." Sound advice for the rest of us.

❤   ❤   ❤

Finish each day and be done with it. You have done what you could. Some blunders and absurdities no doubt crept in; forget them as soon as you can. Tomorrow is a new day; begin it well and serenely and with too high a spirit to be encumbered with your old nonsense.

– Ralph Waldo Emerson –

CHAPTER 21

Laugh your way to good health
Develop your humor skills

L aughter is like a magnet. I find that the more you laugh, the more things seem to get funnier. A strange thing happens on TV every season or so. Ever watch comedy shows? Did you notice that one show spins off to many other shows with the same themes? The TV producers seem to say if one show in a genre is successful, then many more just like it will succeed. If something is good for you, then more of the same is better.

Again, laughter is like a magnet. If you are around it, it's contagious. If you are near it, you are drawn into it. If you hear about it from someone else, you want to be part of it.

I have never stopped laughing, which usually happens when I am either laughing at myself, or chuckling at the events occurring around me. TV writers can never convey on the television screen the humor that occurs every day out in the world we live in. Never. I don't care how hard they try. The need for humor is universal, and built into our DNA. I propose that we all should laugh more, louder, and longer - and do it for no other reason than for our health. With 10 grandchildren calling me up all the time to tell me knock-knock jokes, believe me when I tell you I have to be on my guard at all times. And that's NO joke.

Webster's Dictionary defines humor as "That quality which appeals to a sense of the ludicrous or absurdly incongruous", and "A sudden, unpredictable, or unreasoning inclination", and, "To soothe or content by indulgence." My definition is: "Gut wrenching, side splitting laughter done until my face hurts, my rib cage aches, the smile on my face takes over my entire body, and I have to rush to the bathroom before I explode."

Being in the corporate world for more years than I want to count, I have witnessed first hand a business meeting where the atmosphere is so thick with seriousness-itis that you can cut through the air with a knife. It's not a pretty sight. Yet, when someone takes a chance, bucks the corporate culture, and tells a joke, or a funny anecdote, the room erupts into jovial applause, the tension has been relieved, and the mood has gone from pure doldrums to comic relief, resulting in a freer exchange of ideas, and a more relaxed setting.

There should be a requirement that humor skills be part of the hiring criteria when companies hire their leadership. I tend to respect leaders that use humor to motivate their workers. From my experience in the corporate wars over the years, managers that don't have a good sense of humor seem to be more rigid in their management style than leaders that use comedy to get their point across and move the projects along to their successful conclusion. Managers that are "stick-in-the-mud" types and are considered by the rank and file as "the suits" - are unyielding in their view of the world. Leaders that convey a sense of humor in the workforce are perceived by the people around them as mentors, forward thinkers, confident, self-assured, flexible people and fun to be around.

I suggest that seeing the world tilted just a little "off its axis" is extremely beneficial to your physical, as well as psychological health. Seeing the lighter side of issues and problems helps us defray the stress of the moment, just long enough to gather our thoughts and see the dilemma as it really is. I postulate that we take things much too seriously for our own good.

If we can agree that having a depressing, anxiety-ridden mood is just not fun to be around, could there also be a negative physical effect to having such a personality trait? Looking back into history may be the best answer to the question "is humor and laughter an effective method to curing the ills of the world?" Mark Twain, one of the great literary thinkers of all time, summed it up this way by saying "The human race has only one really effective weapon, and that's laughter. The moment it arises, all our hardnesses yield, all our irritations and resentments slip away, and a sunny spirit takes their place."

Years later, studies have confirmed that people who are extremely depressed had more than 69 percent chance of developing heart disease than those that had a sunny disposition. The thickness of the artery walls occurred more often in very anxious people, according to a study performed between 1996 and 1998. The purely toxic result of holding anger in, being highly anxious, and depressed, translated to hardening of the arteries, high blood pressure, and even death. It is common medical knowledge that during a stressful situation, the adrenal gland releases corticosteroids (cortisol) into the blood stream. The more stress... the more cortisol. Lee Berk, Associate Professor at the University of Loma Linda University School of Medicine, concludes that higher levels of cortisol can impede (or suppress) the immune system. Conversely, he believes that the very act of laughter "can lower cortisol levels, thusly protecting our immune system."

So what benefits are there in adding humor to your skills toolkit, and cutting loose with a little humor? The mechanism of laughter can build intimacy between total strangers, by constructing a common body of understanding between the two parties concerned. Becoming less rigid in our physical mannerisms and our thinking patterns may result in more ways of dealing with problems than "just our way" of thinking.

Good humor and the ability to laugh at the world around you can release the creative juices that allow you to solve problems more easily. This may be that endorphins are released during deep laughter. These types of endorphin are the same kinds that are released after athletes jog for great distance...resulting in what athletes call "runners high." By laughing, you take the top off the "pressure cooker," allowing the body to get back to its normal state more quickly.

Laughter and humor breaks the ice in tense situations, and building rapport through using laughter can be a stress reducer, which has been proven to lower blood pressure, and better control blood flow to the heart muscle. From all the data on the therapeutic benefits of humor now in, humor and laughter are good for the body and soul. And having a personality that integrates humor into your daily routine can actually increase your ability to manage physical, as well as emotional trauma, therefore minimizing the shock of these emotions altogether

Ultimately, laughter can be a tool that helps us better handle the constant changes we are subjected to at home and at work. Laughing forces us to be thrust into the present moment, viewing the absurd and ridiculous for what it is - which IS the absurdity and ridiculousness of it all - then taking control of some the chaos around us...just for a moment, and laughing at it anyway.

Try laughing for a change.

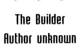

The Builder
Author unknown

AN ELDERLY CARPENTER WAS READY TO RETIRE. HE TOLD HIS EMPLOYER-CONTRACTOR OF HIS PLANS TO LEAVE THE HOUSE BUILDING BUSINESS AND LIVE A MORE LEISURELY LIFE WITH HIS WIFE ENJOYING HIS EXTENDED FAMILY. HE WOULD MISS THE PAYCHECK, BUT HE NEEDED TO RETIRE. THEY COULD GET BY.

THE CONTRACTOR WAS SORRY TO SEE HIS GOOD WORKER GO AND ASKED IF HE COULD BUILD JUST ONE MORE HOUSE AS A PERSONAL FAVOR. THE CARPENTER SAID YES, BUT IN TIME IT WAS EASY TO SEE THAT HIS HEART WAS NOT IN HIS WORK.

HE RESORTED TO SHODDY WORKMANSHIP AND USED IN-FERIOR MATERIALS. IT WAS AN UNFORTUNATE WAY TO END HIS CAREER.

WHEN THE CARPENTER FINISHED HIS WORK AND THE BUILDER CAME TO INSPECT THE HOUSE, THE CONTRACTOR HANDED THE FRONT-DOOR KEY TO THE > CARPENTER.

"THIS IS YOUR HOUSE," HE SAID, "MY GIFT TO YOU." WHAT A SHOCK! WHAT A SHAME! IF HE HAD ONLY KNOWN HE WAS BUILDING HIS OWN HOUSE, HE WOULD HAVE DONE IT ALL SO DIFFERENTLY.

NOW HE HAD TO LIVE IN THE HOME HE HAD BUILT NONE TOO WELL. SO IT IS WITH US. WE BUILD OUR LIVES IN A DISTRACTED WAY, REACTING RATHER THAN ACTING, WILL-ING TO PUT UP LESS THAN THE BEST. AT IMPORTANT POINTS WE DO NOT GIVE THE JOB OUR BEST EFFORT. THEN WITH A SHOCK WE LOOK AT THE SITUATION WE HAVE CREATED AND FIND THAT WE ARE NOW LIVING IN THE HOUSE WE HAVE BUILT. IF WE HAD REALIZED, WE WOULD HAVE DONE IT DIFFERENTLY.

Think of yourself as the carpenter. Think about your house. Each day you hammer a nail, place a board, or erect a wall. Build wisely. It is the only life you will ever build. Even if you live it for only one day more, that day deserves to be lived graciously and with dignity.

The plaque on the wall says, "Life is a do-it-yourself project."

Who could say it more clearly? Your life today is the result of your attitudes and choices in the past. Your life tomorrow will be the result of your attitudes and the choices you make today.

CHAPTER 22

"All I want is some peace of mind"
Meditate - not just medicate

There is a growing group of medical, as well as non-medical groups, and individuals that support the notion of curing human ailments as a "whole", - including the mental, physical, and spiritual self. For example, in the Orient, the mind-body connection has been known for centuries. Most, if not all, religions of the world participate in meditation as a daily ritual of their lifestyle. We in the United States only now fully understand that in a lot of ways, our physical being is intricately linked to our mental and emotional selves.

More and more research is being released daily backing up the claims that meditation, when done on a regular basis, along with exercise, and a solid healthy dietary regiment, might allow you to live a longer and richer life. Current research now postulates that there is a physiological benefit to a continuous and on-going campaign of relaxation. Studies now show that there is a decrease in a hormone called cortisol, which is released by the body as a result of stress, when one meditates on a regular basis. Even though having an ample supply of this hormone is extremely useful in the Fight-or-Flight situation, having this hormone being released into the body on a daily basis, such as the day to day stresses we are under, may actually hinder, or inhibit the body's immune system...thus slowing the repair of damaged tissue.

What was a passing fad in the 1960's and 1970's, during the "Love Generation" has become mainstream in today's stress-laden society. While Transcendental Meditation(tm) and Yoga was practiced by a select few during that time, and looked upon by the "establishment" as being far-fetched and useless, it is now being practiced by the mainstream population and has been endorsed by both the medical community, and the alternative health industry.

Early in the 1990's, Dr. Dean Ornish, who opened the Preventive Medicine Research Center, in Sausalito, California, published an in-depth study stating that someone with heart disease can clear their arteries without using medical drugs if they adopt a pattern of exercise and stress management...which includes meditation. His findings indicate a direct link between on-going stress management techniques and changes in the arteries.

So, how do we meditate? Remembering that this is a "how-to" survival guide, let's jump into it. I'm going to outline a technique I use to release the stresses of the day, which can be done absolutely anywhere you happen to be which allows you a little peace, quiet, and solitude. I will emphasize that this meditation requires you to close your eyes while doing the exercise...so don't try this on the freeway (I have always found it very difficult to drive with my eyes shut).

For most of us (me included), there is never enough time to do the things we need to do during a 24-hour period, let alone learn a new technique. But you may find out, as I have, that by doing this exercise, and slowing down for a moment during the busy day, to reflect on what is really important in life, this meditative technique adds quality to your day...and in turn might add quantity to your life as well.

The "10 to 1 and 3 to 1 Countdown" technique has been taught by Jose Silva for many years throughout the World, in his Silva International, Inc. Basic Lecture Series 101 thru 404 courses. I would suggest that anyone wishing to hone their meditation techniques... or learn them from scratch, should purchase his book "The Silva Method" at your local bookseller. If you desire more hands-on training, his organization can provide you with local instructors trained in teaching the technique. Taking two days out of your busy schedule will be well worth the time - to learn this valuable tool.

10 to 1 Countdown

Find a comfortable chair to sit in, and while sitting, relax your entire body. Take off your shoes if you like. Tighten your toes into the carpet (if there is carpet under you). Don't tighten up your body. Any position that is comforting to you is the right position. Now close your eyes.

Take in a few breaths, breathing deeper with each one. Try to take in enough to fill your chest cavity. As you are taking in clean, energizing air, visualize that you are pulling in positive energy around you.

As you exhale, and while slowly and silently saying the number "10 deeper" three times, visualize the number 10 and see yourself relaxed. See the tension leaving your body. As you relax, you will feel your body going into a deepened state of relaxation.

Inhale, and as you do so, visualize a huge wave of total relaxation flowing over every inch of your body...starting at the top of your head flowing onto and over your feet and running out onto the floor around you.

As you exhale, and while slowly and silently saying and visualizing the number "9 deeper" three times, visualize the letter 9 and see yourself relaxed. See the tension leaving your body. As you relax, you will feel your body going into a deepened state of relaxation...deeper and deeper, deeper than you were before.

Inhale, and as you do so, visualize a huge wave of total relaxation flowing over every inch of your body...starting at the top of your head flowing onto and over your feet and running out onto the floor around you. Feel the waves of relaxation seeping into your skin, and into your blood stream. Going deeper and deeper...deeper than you have been before. Sense all the stress leaving your body.

Repeat the above steps until you reach the number 1...saying at each lower number that you are going deeper, and deeper...deeper than you have been before, profoundly deeper than you have been before.

As you mentally say the word "Zero", daydream that you are at a calm, wonderfully peaceful place you know. It could be a lake you visited when you were a child, or a favorite vacation spot you went to in the not too distant past. Dream about whatever place you feel totally free from the daily stresses of life. Taste, smell, feel, and sense how it "felt" to be totally safe, secure, and at peace with the world.

While at this secret "hiding place," say to yourself mentally "Every day in every way, I am getting better and better...better than I was before."

After savoring the relaxation of being in this magical healing place, slowly count forward from 1 to 3, saying at each number that "when I finally open my eyes, I will feel wide awake, stress free, healed, and better than before."

When you reach the count of 4, repeat this phrase "when I finally open my eyes, I will feel wide awake, stress free, healed, and better than before."

Reaching the count of Five, open your eyes, take a deep breath, and feel all the stress gone, feeling better and better, better than you felt before.

I would suggest that you read the above instructions a number of times, then perform the meditation and see how it feels to you. After you have done it for a few days, it will become easier and easier to do. You might want to take a tape recorder and record the instructions, then play the tape back when you have a few minutes to spare. Make a point of taking a number of stress breaks during the day. I find that I do a shortened session, but counting from 3 to 1 - before I go into a meeting that may be stressful. Another trick is to do the countdown before you make a difficult telephone call. You will find that the more you practice, the faster you will become relaxed, and the more often you are relaxed, the better you feel, and the less stress you are under. Once you become proficient, just by saying the word Relax, you will be relaxed.

Another fun thing to do is to find props to use to enlist relaxation. When I am in an elevator, as I descend from one floor to the next, I use the descending numbers to remind me of the countdown technique. I have been known to do the 10 to 1 and 3 to 1 countdown technique as a passenger in a car, or a plane. It works wonders.

Using the 10 to 1 and 3 to 1 technique once per day is wonderful, twice per day is outstanding, and three times per day is fantastic. Utilizing this meditation on a regular basis will provide you with a tool for the reconnection of your body, mind and soul by removing the stressful distractions thrust upon us all on a daily basis. Giving ourselves permission to "relax", just for a moment, may be the greatest medicine available, and it's free for the taking.

❤ ❤ ❤

Take time every day to do something silly
- Philipa Walker -

C H A P T E R **23**

"Think yourself to perfect health"
Techniques for visualization of a successful recovery

I see what you mean." "Can you imagine how he feels?" Have you ever watched a stage Hypnotist telling his subject to "Visualize yourself on a beach - drink in hand, looking at a calm blue sea?" The most compelling statement that describes how truly powerful the mind really is can be stated by the following:

A picture is worth a thousand words

What if you could, by harnessing immense power and imagination, tap into the healing forces lying just under the surface of your mind and using this power, to heal what ails you? Would that be the most awesome tool we all have to conquer both physical and mental diseases running loose in the world today?

We are all famous for visualizing the worst of a situation. When you were young and single, did you not sweat before you went out on a date and said things like "I know he or she won't like me" ...to find out later, that you were exactly what he or she was expecting. When you are about to go into a job interview, you don't think about all the positive things you have to offer the employer, but instead, you think of all the things they may find wrong with your qualifications. You sweat all the small things in life. Mark Twain said, "I am an old man and have known a great many troubles - but most of them never happened." How many of our ailments have turned out to be "in our head?" A doctor once informed me that if you think you are healthy, you are right...and if you think you are unhealthy...you are also right. Why not think that we are healthy, happy people? It's a lot more fun and may just benefit you in ways you can't imagine.

Before you can fully appreciate the techniques that I am about to show you, we need to understand the difference between the acts of seeing, visualization (to visualize), and imagination (to imagine).

Seeing is a physical action performed by using your eyes to witness the world around you. The eyes see, then the mind takes those signals, turns them into data, which the brain then interprets based on past knowledge, experiences, and training.

Visualization (to visualize) is the mind digging back into the brain's database of past "actual" events and recalling what some thing, some one, or some place actually looked like. The act of visualization is not as vivid an image as physically seeing something first hand. But visualization does produce extremely realistic images of past events. Just close your eyes and visualize a past pleasurable event in your life. If your skill at visualization is trained, the event can be profound, and the reenactment of that event will be as close to the actual event in intensity, as if you were there.

Imagination (to imagine) is an extremely creative process, whereby you invent an image in your mind...even

🖤 🖤 🖤

Life's like a game of poker: If you don't put any in the pot, there won't be any to take out
- Moms Mabley -

though that image never existed before. An example of this would be if you wanted to be rich, and then imagined yourself being rich. You were never rich, are not rich now...but desire to be rich in the future. That's imagination. If you were rich before, lost your wealth, you could then visualize yourself being rich again, because you have been a rich person before. Your brain's database pulls out already-stored information, which you then draw on to build a movie screen to view yourself being rich again. The same analogy can be used for visualizing optimum health and vitality. You were once healthy, full of life, youthful and exuberant. Since your brain stored all that information before, you can draw on that experience by using visualization techniques to be that way again.

Using the techniques for getting into a relaxed state of being by performing the 10 to 1 and 3 to 1 relaxation method outlined in the previous chapter, you are now ready to learn how to use your mind to perform guided imagery to visualize yourself healing meditatively. The key to success to any meditative practice is that of truly wanting and believing that healing will take place and your expectation that it will happen for you.

There arc numerous methods, and techniques, for applying guided imagery, and one may be more effective FOR YOU than others. Take it upon yourself to learn about the different methods, and organizations, that offer guided imagery training. More and more hospitals and physicians are utilizing guided imagery, including audio tapes, with their patients, because they now understand it may make a profound impact on the quality of care, and of life inside, as well as outside, of the operating room - as well as later when the patient goes home to recuperate and to resume his or her normal duties of living.

While in the relaxed mode, visualize the cells of your body being inflamed, then gradually view them morphing into healthy vibrant cells. Visualize the healthy cells chasing after the inflamed and damaged cells, consuming the unhealthy cells and becoming pure. See your entire body as a clean, pure, healthy, vibrant, and happy place. See your body as a temple of pure health and vitality.

While in the relaxed mode, visualize the cells of your heart muscle being inflamed, then gradually view them morphing into healthy vibrant cells. Visualize the healthy cells chasing after the inflamed and damaged cells, consuming the unhealthy cells and becoming pure. View the arteries of your heart as they are now, clogged up and the blood stream not pure and the blood not flowing smoothly. Now visualize you pouring a bottle of healthy artery cleaner into the heart muscle, and view before you the arteries becoming clean of clogs, pure, and flowing better than the arteries have flowed before. See your entire body as a clean, pure, healthy, vibrant, and happy place. See your body as a temple of pure health and vitality.

While in the relaxed mode, visualize the cells of your entire body being inflamed, then gradually view them morphing into healthy vibrant cells. Visualize the healthy cells chasing after the inflamed and damaged cells, consuming the unhealthy cells and becoming pure. View the cells as they are now, un-energized, weak, and not pure. and not working at optimal efficiency. Now visualize yourself opening a bottle of pure cellular energy and witness yourself consuming the entire bottle. Visualize the transformation taking affect instantly in every part

❤ ❤ ❤

The truth is not what hurts; it's the denial
- Kelly Imber -

of your body from the hair on the top of your head, to the tips of your toes, cleaning and re-vitalizing every molecule in your body. See your entire body as a clean, pure, healthy, vibrant, and happy place. See your body as a temple of pure health and vitality.

Have fun with the exercises and don't take them too seriously. Change the routine every time you mediate. If I am in a stressful situation, such as work, I go to my relaxed mode, then visualize little "pacman" type of healthy cells gobbling up the stress cells. After awhile, you can do a standing meditation while waiting for a street light to change, or while sitting in a conference room waiting for a meeting to begin. Doing it before a perceived stressful situation builds up an immune system - not allowing the stress to occur in the first place.

At the end of every meditative session, say to yourself the following: "I am getting better and better...better than I was before, healthier and healthier and healthier." Your body will respond accordingly. Every meditation session should have three sections: (1) identify the blocked or damaged area, (2) psychically SEE the area of disease being repaired, and (3) seeing and believing the area, as well as your entire body, totally cured. These techniques really do work, but the rate and degree of your healing depends on your attitude and readiness to be healthy, happy and whole.

❤   ❤   ❤

~Jack Riemer, Houston Chronicle, February 10, 2001~

The following true story, written in 1995 by Jack Riemer , has been circulating around the Internet for years. Even though you might be familiar with the story, it may be time to reexamine it's powerful message

On Nov. 18, 1995, Itzhak Perlman, the violinist, came on stage to give a concert at Avery Fisher Hall at Lincoln Center in New York City. If you have ever been to a Perlman concert, you know that getting on stage is no small achievement for him. He was stricken with polio as a child, and so he has braces on both legs and walks with the aid of two crutches. To see him walk across the stage one step at a time, painfully and slowly, is an awesome sight. He walks painfully, yet majestically, until he reaches his chair. Then he sits down, slowly, puts his crutches on the floor, undoes the clasps on his legs, tucks one foot back and extends the other foot forward.

Then he bends down and picks up the violin, puts it under his chin, nods to the conductor and proceeds to play.

By now, the audience is used to this ritual. They sit quietly while he makes his way across the stage to his chair. They remain reverently silent while he undoes the clasps on his legs. They wait until he is ready to play. But this time, something went wrong. Just as he finished the first few bars, one of the strings on his violin broke. You could hear it snap - it went off

like gunfire across the room. There was no mistaking what that sound meant.

There was no mistaking what he had to do.

PEOPLE WHO WERE THERE THAT NIGHT THOUGHT TO THEMSELVES: *"WE FIGURED THAT HE WOULD HAVE TO GET UP, PUT ON THE CLASPS AGAIN, PICK UP THE CRUTCHES AND LIMP HIS WAY OFF STAGE - TO EITHER FIND ANOTHER VIOLIN OR ELSE FIND ANOTHER STRING FOR THIS ONE."*

BUT HE DIDN'T. INSTEAD, HE WAITED A MOMENT, CLOSED HIS EYES AND THEN SIGNALED THE CONDUCTOR TO BEGIN AGAIN. THE ORCHESTRA BEGAN, AND HE PLAYED FROM WHERE HE HAD LEFT OFF. AND HE PLAYED WITH SUCH PASSION AND SUCH POWER AND SUCH PURITY AS THEY HAD NEVER HEARD BEFORE.

OF COURSE, ANYONE KNOWS THAT IT IS IMPOSSIBLE TO PLAY A SYMPHONIC WORK WITH JUST THREE STRINGS. I KNOW THAT, AND YOU KNOW THAT, BUT THAT NIGHT ITZHAK PERLMAN REFUSED TO KNOW THAT. YOU COULD SEE HIM MODULATING, CHANGING, RECOMPOSING THE PIECE IN HIS HEAD. AT ONE POINT, IT SOUNDED LIKE HE WAS DE-TUNING THE STRINGS TO GET NEW SOUNDS FROM THEM THAT THEY HAD NEVER MADE BEFORE.

WHEN HE FINISHED, THERE WAS AN AWESOME SILENCE IN THE ROOM. AND THEN PEOPLE ROSE AND CHEERED. THERE WAS AN EXTRAORDINARY OUTBURST OF APPLAUSE FROM EVERY CORNER OF THE AUDITORIUM. WE WERE ALL ON OUR FEET, SCREAMING AND CHEERING, DOING EVERY-THING WE COULD TO SHOW HOW MUCH WE APPRECIATED WHAT HE HAD DONE.

HE SMILED, WIPED THE SWEAT FROM THIS BROW, RAISED HIS BOW TO QUIET US, AND THEN HE SAID - NOT BOAST-FULLY, BUT IN A QUIET, PENSIVE, REVERENT TONE - *"YOU KNOW, SOMETIMES IT IS THE ARTIST'S TASK TO FIND OUT HOW MUCH MUSIC YOU CAN STILL MAKE WITH WHAT YOU HAVE LEFT."*

WHAT A POWERFUL LINE THAT IS. IT HAS STAYED IN MY MIND EVER SINCE I HEARD IT. AND WHO KNOWS? PERHAPS THAT IS THE DEFINITION OF LIFE - NOT JUST FOR ARTISTS

BUT FOR ALL OF US. HERE IS A MAN WHO HAS PREPARED ALL HIS LIFE TO MAKE MUSIC ON A VIOLIN OF FOUR STRINGS, WHO, ALL OF A SUDDEN, IN THE MIDDLE OF A CONCERT, FINDS HIMSELF WITH ONLY THREE STRINGS; SO HE MAKES MUSIC WITH THREE STRINGS, AND THE MUSIC HE MADE THAT NIGHT WITH JUST THREE STRINGS WAS MORE BEAUTI-FUL, MORE SACRED, MORE MEMORABLE, THAN ANY THAT HE HAD EVER MADE BEFORE, WHEN HE HAD FOUR STRINGS.

SO, PERHAPS OUR TASK IN THIS SHAKY, FAST-CHANGING, BEWILDERING WORLD IN WHICH WE LIVE IS TO MAKE MU-SIC, AT FIRST WITH ALL THAT WE HAVE, AND THEN, WHEN THAT IS NO LONGER POSSIBLE, TO MAKE MUSIC WITH WHAT WE HAVE LEFT.

C H A P T E R 24

To succeed - don't do the things that make you fail

I want to introduce a new concept into your mindset. There are literally hundreds of well-respected teachers in the world that give us all the ways that you can be successful in your lives. Be it success in money, love, health, finance, raising children, car racing, physical fitness, and so on and so on. There is a one billion-dollar industry in America on Self Help remedies, of which this book proudly falls into.

The concept that I am about to present is so simple, it probably has not been thought of before, which goes to show you that there are still great ideas out there that need to be thought of.

I was brought up to believe that if I did all the RIGHT things in life, I would live forever, be extremely happy, physically fit, financially set and morally right. Oh, and let's not forget ethically straight. But things are not as they seem. The problem with all these wonderful things is that the only thing I was told was that to get to these exalted spots I had to be successful. There were no road maps to follow.

Well, I mean to tell you, I really tried. I do believe for the most part that I am successful in most of the important things in life... but how I got there was, at times, REALLY hard. I focused very hard on doing the right things all the time, which put enormous pressure (and stress) on me. I was following a tried and true way of becoming successful. It should have worked...due to the lessons, which had been handed down over the generations and written about in all the great motivational and success help books.

I believe I have found the fly in the ointment to these great books. They all start you on your journey from ground zero. Meaning they presume you know nothing and they are going to teach you everything you need to be successful. I believe we all have in us a core desire and a core set of talents that make us already successful. We just need to maintain our level of success, get focused, reduce stress, and build on our accomplishments.

To that end, I present a different, and I think a better way of looking at success, and in turn lowering your stress level. Here it is: "To be successful - Don't do the things that make you fail." Let me say it again so it really sinks in. "To be REALLY successful - Don't do the things that make you fail."

Let me explain this concept with a number of examples that I think will drive home the true value of this way of thinking. Let's say that you are at a street corner, wanting to cross the street. The light turns green and you have the legal right to cross the street, but you see that a concrete delivery truck is not about to stop and is in the process of running "his" red light. You say what the hell, I have the right to cross the street, and by golly, I will cross the street. SPLAT. You're a goner. You were DEAD right. To put it in the context of this essay, "you did the thing that made you fail."

I know that was a pretty extreme example. Here's another...softer example. I am on a weight control program to drop some un-needed pounds. I know what foods I should eat, and in what quantities to consume, to reach my ideal size and weight for my body frame. But I just have to eat that chocolate candy bar. If I consume the bar, knowing full well it is not in the food groups I am allowed to pick from, then I am "doing the thing that makes me fail," and consequently, because of my action, will gain weight instead of lose weight.

Let's take another example to illustrate this idea. You are at work, and in a public setting with your boss and a bunch of co-workers, - say standing around the water cooler. There is a discussion going on and all of a sudden, your boss blurts out something that is absolutely NOT TRUE about you. You have three choices: Confront him/her in front of the other people, keep your lips sealed (stressful), or wait till you are both alone and bring up the misinformation to him behind closed doors, strongly suggesting that he send out a memo with the corrected information to the group forthwith.

Remembering the new ethos of "never do the thing that make you fail" may stop you from showing the world how wrong he/she was by bringing up his/her lack of knowledge on that subject by doing it in the group setting. (This action may also embarrass your boss and bosses tend not to forget...particularly around promotion time). Keeping silent can only let the event stay internal in you until it boils over at some future time. You may consider telling him/her your feelings in private. Remember you are already successful, but just remember: "To succeed, don't do the things in life that make you fail." Try it.

❤ ❤ ❤

Don't step on the land mines of life
- Brad Henson -

❤   ❤   ❤

Contributed by: Kelly Imber via the Internet
Original author unknown
A VERY GOOD MOTIVATION FOR ONESELF

A WELL-KNOWN SPEAKER STARTED OFF HIS SEMINAR BY HOLDING UP A $20 BILL. IN THE ROOM OF 200, HE ASKED, "WHO WOULD LIKE THIS $20 BILL?" HANDS STARTED GOING UP. HE SAID, "I AM GOING TO GIVE THIS $20 TO ONE OF YOU BUT FIRST LET ME DO THIS." HE PROCEEDED TO CRUMPLE THE DOLLAR BILL UP. HE THEN ASKED, "WHO STILL WANTS IT?" STILL THE HANDS WERE UP IN THE AIR. "WELL," HE REPLIED, "WHAT IF I DO THIS?" AND HE DROPPED IT ON THE GROUND AND STARTED TO GRIND IT INTO THE FLOOR WITH HIS SHOE. HE PICKED IT UP, NOW ALL CRUMPLED AND DIRTY. "NOW WHO STILL WANTS IT?" STILL THE HANDS WENT INTO THE AIR.

"MY FRIENDS, YOU HAVE ALL LEARNED A VERY VALUABLE LESSON. NO MATTER WHAT I DID TO THE MONEY, YOU STILL WANTED IT BECAUSE IT DID NOT DECREASE IN VALUE. IT WAS STILL WORTH $20. MANY TIMES IN OUR LIVES, WE ARE DROPPED, CRUMPLED, AND GROUND INTO THE DIRT BY THE DECISIONS WE MAKE AND THE CIRCUMSTANCES THAT COME OUR WAY. WE FEEL AS THOUGH WE ARE WORTHLESS.

"BUT NO MATTER WHAT HAS HAPPENED OR WHAT WILL HAPPEN, YOU WILL NEVER LOSE YOUR VALUE. YOU ARE SPECIAL - DON'T EVER FORGET IT! NEVER LET YESTERDAY'S DISAPPOINTMENTS OVERSHADOW TOMORROW'S DREAMS."

CHAPTER 25

"Lets get Physical"
Benefits of exercise and your heart

E xercising is like paying, or not paying, the house hold utility bills. What happens if you don't pay the phone bill? Try calling up your phone company and say that you have decided to "not" pay the bill this month...and see if they will buy it. I don't think so! What is more likely to happen is that one morning, you get out of bed, pick up the phone to place a necessary call, BAM, the phone is dead. There is this silence at the other end. Think of it in financial terms. If you don't invest a few dollars in a solid, and long-term investment program, you won't have financial freedom in your old age. The same is true with exercise. If you don't take time out EVERY DAY to exercise, you won't have the physical freedom from disease in the "Golden years" to go along with the financial freedom you have worked so hard for. It's as simple as that.

Do you brush you teeth, take a shower, comb you hair, and put on clothes in the morning - before you go to work or school? I hope so. Then, why not make it a point to do a little exercise, every day? "I am so busy, I don't have time to go the gym." Or "With all the stuff I have to do at work, I have no time to add anything else to my schedule" is heard in homes, and workplaces, around the world.

Like paying your bills, or doing proper hygiene, exercise has to be part of your daily routine. My old gym coach in High School constantly told us that exercise gives you a "natural high." Looking back on how I felt after running 20 or so miles up and down the hills of Chatsworth, California after school every day...I can now see what he meant. I felt invigorated, rejuvenated, and refreshed. Exercising on a regular basis allows the body to rid itself of toxins, and I for one feel great after working out on the Bowflex(tm), swimming, or going for a strenuous walk. It has been proven, through a study at the University of Southern California, that going for a 15 minute walk resulted in reduction of bodily tension equal to or greater than taking a strong tranquilizer.

It's a great return on investment, meaning that the benefits far outweigh the cost. From a stress related point-of-view, getting away from the house, office, boss, kids, parents, wife, husband, boyfriend, girlfriend, and co-workers for a while is worth every minute of exercising you do. You may be asking the same question I did before I got SERIOUS about making the time to exercise: "Everyone says you need to exercise, but no one tells you why." What's in it for me? What's my return-on-investment?

The answer up front, plain and simple is this. All of the following is important to you, based on your own needs, desires, and wants. The first, and most important to me was a reduced risk of having another heart attack. When I exercise, I have more energy, and less stress in my life than when I don't. Many times I will be in a situation where I feel stress coming on, and I say to my wife..."I am going for a long walk (exercise)." When I return, I feel stress free, I have a better ability to concentrate, reduced anxiety and hostility toward the person (or event) that caused me to be upset before my walk, and a better disposition (elevated mood) than I did before. I also find that after I go for a long walk, I sleep better. If you exercise on a regular basis, your body weight is more apt to be properly controlled, and your body might be apt to look "firmer" than if you were a couch potato.

From a purely medical perspective, there are solid reasons that exercising is beneficial to your heart and your health. Viscous, or sticky blood, elevated blood pressure, and narrowing of the arteries is a physical reaction to increased levels of stress, which ultimately reduces the blood flow to the heart. There have been cases reported that show irregular heartbeats, and heart attacks can be caused by psychological stress.

Medical studies have documented positive results about people who take the time about out their busy schedule to exercise regularly. One such benefit is that folks who exercise regularly are more apt to take in stride daily stresses over inactive, non-exercising individuals. One study indicated that physical symptoms, (chest pain or joint pain) are more likely to show up in 37 percent of non-exercisers.

There have been numerous occasions when I am angry for some reason, my wife noticing this may say intuitively, "Brad - go for a walk." Being a recovering Type "A" person, she knows that she must force me to take ACTION. She also knows that this action will result in me working out my stress, thus reducing the chance that I may blow a gasket...figuratively and physically.

If you have had a bad day at the office, working out at the gym, or going for a long walk, or performing other types of exercise, may be the perfect alternative over that brought on by the Fight or Flight reaction to stress our ancestors experienced by hunting, or being chased by wild animals. Exercise is a much better solution than fighting a co-worker, or tangling, or fleeing from a wild animal (whether they be man or beast). When I am under a stressful situation, (like what happens a hundred times per day at work), my blood pressure increases, I find myself breathing faster than normal, and my muscles get very tense. According to Edward A. Charlesworth, PHD, and Ronald G. Natham, PHD in their book, *Stress Management - a Comprehensive Guide to Wellness*, the "body pours stored sugars and fats into the bloodstream."

But if you ask what types, how much, how hard, or how long you should exercise, can you then develop immunity toward heart disease? In the exercise industry, these are called duration, frequency, and intensity. The other important factors in obtaining good health are aerobic activity, muscular strengthening, and flexibility.

According to the medical community, the frequency should be a minimum of three times per week. The duration of your exercise program should be between 20 and 30 minutes per section. The last factor to consider is the intensity of the exercise being done. I used to measure the intensity of my treadmill time using this simple technique. If I could walk and talk at the same time, then I was properly doing the exercise correctly, and getting the most benefits. If I can't perform the "talk test", then I know I am working out too vigorously.

The American Council on Exercise (ACE) indicates that aerobic activity assists the lungs and heart muscle to reduce body fat by increasing caloric expenditure.

After my heart attack, I was fearful of getting back into the routine of heavy exercise. I was running very long distances at the time, and to be quite frank about it, I was fearful of having another heart attack by overdoing myself and exercising too hard. After getting the okay from the Cardiologist to start working out again, I proceeded to start a walking program. My first motivation was to use the walking as a way to force myself to relax. Walking by myself afforded me the opportunity to release the stresses of the day, and to just spend time "thinking." This time was a mental release and time to sort things out, and clear my mind of all the clutter of the day's activity.

The added benefit to my walking program was that my heart muscle was getting stronger and stronger. My doctor explained to me that a well-conditioned heart muscle becomes more powerful, hence more efficient and consequently beats slower. Because I was exercising the heart muscle, it became better at pumping blood throughout the body. Have you ever noticed that your car runs much more smoothly after you arrive home from a long road trip? How about after you get into the car first thing in the morning, after the car has been sitting out in the cold weather all night? Notice how rough the engine runs. It's the same thing with the heart before and after exercise.

I was skeptical about the benefits of exercise on my blood pressure readings. So I did the following test. The first thing I did was record my blood pressure and note the systolic and diastolic numbers. Then I went out and exercised for a while (after I got permission from my Cardiologist). After completing my exercising, I allowed my body to "cool down", I retook my blood pressure again. You may notice, as I did, that the numbers are lower. I guess the old adage of "Either use it or lose it" makes a lot of sense.

Flexibility can be achieved by stretching. If you live in a house and/or have a yard, there is always yard work or housework to do. Try mowing the lawn, bending down and pulling weeds, raking the leaves, taking out the metal trash cans from the garage to the curb...without placing them on rollers, but instead pulling or pushing them and see how much sweat you can produce. Talk you wife into keeping the kids home from school for a day. I guarantee you will be exercised to the max and feel the "burn" by the end the end of the day. Who needs a health club to go to when you have a workout program built into the responsibility of being a dad or a mom?

The bottom line to the flexibility, aerobic and muscular strengthening program is two little, but very powerful words. TAKE ACTION. Get off your rear-end, and take advantage of what you have at hand to make the exercise program work for you. Doing exercise at the end of a busy day at the office is a lot better way of burning off stress than doing drugs, or alcohol, with greater benefits - giving you a tool to manage stress.

❦   ❦   ❦

Zen Master
Contributed by Beth Henson via the Internet
Original author unknown

So the Zen master steps up to the hot dog stand and says: "Make me one with everything." The hot dog vendor fixes a hot dog and hands it to the Zen master, who pays with a $20 bill. The hot dog vendor puts the bill in the cash register and closes the drawer. "Where's my change?" asks the Zen master. And the hot dog vendor responds, "Change must come from within."

CHAPTER 26

Clean your "garage"

Do you ever notice people's garages? Beth and I go
for walks throughout the neighborhood on a regular
basis...to pick up a few groceries at the local mart, or to
visit a number of cats that live along the way. You can't
help but notice the homes as you pass by them. I tend to
look at the garages and wonder if the condition of the
garage reflects somehow the level of organization, and
stress level that the owner lives under. I am not a certi-
fied psychologist, but have been around the block a number of times, and do believe there is a correlation between cleanliness of garages and one's stress level.

It may have to do with "holding on" to things...in this
case "stuff". I know I hold on to things a lot longer than
Beth does. I also have more stress than she does. Hello.
The comedian George Carlin has a great skit that he has
been performing on stage for years and years. He says
that when people get their first house, they have a little
"stuff" and then they get a bigger house, and guess what?
They move their "stuff" from the little place to the bigger
place and now they fill up the bigger house with MORE
STUFF. This goes on and on till they burst from the over-
load of the stuff they have been carrying around with
them over the years.

I was like that, particularly with clothes. I have gained and lost a ton of weight over the years, and because of this, have bought clothes to fit when I was thinner, and when I was fatter. My closet looked like a department store clothes rack. The only thing missing was the plastic size indicators between the different sizes. We have a large walk-in closet at the house and I took up a lot more space than Beth needed to hang her clothes.

Does the stuff in the garage and the stuff in the house represent some deep rooted issue that I may be harboring? Possibly! Over the last year or so, I have tossed out ALL the clothes in my closet that did not properly fit.

I then proceeded to spend a lot of time in the garage getting rid of all the "stuff" that I have been carrying around with me for years. Boy, does it feel good to throw things away. I finally realized that there was NO reason to keep things that I NEVER use any more. After the garage cleaning was over, I journeyed into the office, turned on the computer, and started to clean out all the "saved mail" that I had been collecting over the last year or two. I am now working on removing any unread documents that I will never look at again that lie unopened on my hard drive. Wow, look at the money I am saving by doing needed hard drive clean up, and not needing to buy a bigger hard drive!!

I have started to take it one step further and have examined some negative feelings about people in my life and dealt with those issues straight on. It's amazing how good I have been feeling and how "clean my garage is" now that I have gotten control of this part of my life. I am not quite there yet, but I know I am going in the right direction.

♥   ♥   ♥

Cleanliness is next to Godliness
- Old Hebrew saying -

Try cleaning your garage and see if there is any other "stuff" you can toss out. See if there are angry or bad feelings about a family member, or someone at work that you have been holding onto far longer than you should. The reality is: The person you are mad at probably doesn't even know you are mad at them. The only one you are hurting by holding on to the "stuff" called anger is you. Get rid of it. You may find something you thought was lost forever a long time ago...peace of mind.

He who does not get fun and enjoyment out of every day...
needs to reorganize his life
- George Mathew Adams -

C H A P T E R 27

Get to know, and like, the child within you

I would like to share with you the following story I re
ceived from someone via the Internet the other day.
The author is unknown but the message drives home
the fact that we adults take life way too seriously. I read
this every once in a while...just to keep a clear perspective on life.

Adult Resignation

I am hereby officially tendering my resignation
as an adult. I have decided I would like to accept
the responsibilities of an 8-year-old again. I want
to go to McDonald's and think that it's a four star
restaurant. I want to sail sticks across a fresh mud
puddle and make ripples with rocks. I want to
think M&Ms are better than money because you
can eat them. I want to lie under a big oak tree
and run a lemonade stand with my friends on a
hot summer's day. I want to return to a time when
life was colors, multiplication tables, and nurs-
ery rhymes, but that didn't bother you, because
you didn't know what you didn't know and you
didn't care. All you knew was to be happy because you were blissfully unaware of all the things

that should make you worried or upset. I want to think the world is fair. That everyone is honest and good. I want to believe that anything is possible. I want to be oblivious to the complexities of life and be overly excited by the little things again. I want to live simple again. I don't want my day to consist of computer crashes, mountains of paperwork, depressing news, how to survive more days in the month than there is money in the bank, doctor bills, gossip, illness, and loss of loved ones. I want to believe in the power of smiles, hugs, a kind word, truth, justice, peace, dreams, the imagination, mankind, and making angels in the snow. So....here's my checkbook and my car keys, my credit card bills and my 401K statements. I am officially resigning from adulthood. And if you want to discuss this further, you'll have to catch me first, cause, "Tag! You're it."

I just love that story. It's really cool. So there!

Do you ever wonder why kids never get stressed out like we adults do...I mean to the point of succumbing to a stress related disease. Children seem to have a deep well of energy, vitality, and an abundance of fun to draw from and it seems to never end. What is their secret that we can use to keep our stress level in check? Perhaps it's that they don't take things too seriously. Or maybe it's that they laugh more at the stupidest things for no apparent reason, or maybe they just know that things are not as serious as they appear to be.

Sure, when the young man stopped by one night a number of years ago to pick up our daughter, Kimberly, for their first date, I am sure Ben, the young man, was REALLY stressed out. I could see the pimples pop out one-by-one on his young face as we were standing in the living room grilling him on what his intent was to be with our daughter. Did he have insurance on the car he was driving? Was his license current? Where was he really taking her for the evening?...and it couldn't be as simple as the movie. Stress. You want to see stress, then you should have been there that night. It is a rite of passage for young people to withstand the rampages of the parents on their daughter's first car date.

We are happy to say that Ben withstood our bursts of emotionalism...and dated our daughter for a number of years after that night. We are proud to say that he still calls us "mom and dad" and has remained part of the family. I look back on that incident and wonder how wigged out and stressed we looked to these wonderful young people.

Besides the occasional stressful situation like I have mentioned above, young people have the uncanny ability to have fun...at a moment's notice. I try to never forget to be "child like"...once per day. When given lemons, I make lemonade, when it rains, I stand outside and marvel at how wonderful the world is, and that I am in it. When I am with my Grandchildren, I get down on all "fours" and become the best horse I can be to the cowboys and cowgirls in my life.

When Beth and I visited New Zealand on holiday last year, we got really good news from back home about a condo we had purchased in Hawaii that had just closed escrow. We were so excited we could hardly maintain our excitement over the great news we had just received. The thrill was so wonderful, I did an Irish jig where I stood...right in front of a Burger King restaurant...and everyone watching me must have thought I was crazy. I didn't care. I allowed my child to come out and enjoyed every moment of it.

The point is to get to know - and like - the child inside you. See what a difference it makes in your overall health. It may become a habit that you refuse to give up.

Learn to give yourself permission to play again...so there.

❤   ❤   ❤

So get a few laughs and do the best you can
– Will Rogers –

CHAPTER 28

The parable of the old alley cat and the young kitten
Live a passionate life

I was listening to a tape by Wayne Dyer the other day and he told a very funny story, which, I feel has major relevance to reducing stress in our daily lives. It goes something like this. There was this old alley cat and this very young kitten. The young kitten was trying to catch his tail in his mouth. The old alley cat asked what the young kitten was doing. The young kitten said to the old alley cat that he had just gotten back from attending cat psychology school and had learned the meaning of success. Being the old and wise alley cat, and being somewhat of a world traveler himself, the old cat was intrigued by what the younger cat may have learned in cat psychology school.

The young cat said he learned that success was in a cat's tail. He also learned that if a cat were to catch his tail in his mouth...he would have a LOCK on success. The older cat said that was very interesting. The old cat stated that he had been all over the world, in most of the famous back alleys of the most beautiful cities on the planet, by traveling on trains, trucks, and freighters. He, too, had learned that success was at the end of a cat's tail, but, unlike the lesson learned by the younger kitten in cat psychology school, the old cat came to this conclusion (by himself?). If a cat were to do the things that made him or her happy and not worry about chasing after success, success would follow him/her wherever they went.

Why do I mention this parable in a book on stress reduction? Because if you are like I was, and like other competitive-driven human beings, we tend to chase after success like the young cat chasing after his tail. This leads to enormous amounts of unneeded stress on our physical as well as emotional systems and in my case led to a "crash and burn" scenario called a heart attack.

I recommend that we take the approach of the older and wiser cat in doing the things that we are passionately in love with, to fill up our daily lives. Did you ever notice that when you do the things that make you really happy, time "flies?" You look at your watch or clock after you have been totally engulfed in your passion and notice that the hours have flown by. An example of this for me is when I draw, or write, or spend time with my wife, kids or grandkids. I lose all track of time, place, and things around me and am amazed at how much time has gone by when I look at my watch after participating in these activities.

I suggest that for your future survival, you learn very quickly what really turns you on in your own personal life. If you had a magic wand... and could make anything happen in your life that would keep you not only busy, but passionately living a no-limit kind of life...what would it be? I suggest that you might use the three by five card goal setting procedure outlined in this book to set a goal of doing what your HEART tells you YOU should be doing. In my case and while I was in the hospital (with heart monitors attached to me and nurses hanging

When something (an affliction) happens to you,
you either let it defeat you, or you defeat it.
- Rosalind Russell -

over me), I concluded that the only way for me to survive and thrive was to stop selling IBM typewriters and start to live a passionate life. Think about what you wanted to do when you were a small boy or girl. Think about your dreams before your parents started to express their opinions on what you should do or be when you grew up. Listen to the "voice" inside you and you will be amazed at what you will hear.

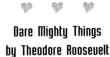

Dare Mighty Things
by Theodore Roosevelt

IN THE BATTLE OF LIFE, IT IS NOT THE CRITIC WHO COUNTS; NOR THE ONE WHO POINTS OUT HOW THE STRONG PERSON STUMBLED, OR WHERE THE DOER OF A DEED COULD HAVE DONE BETTER.

THE CREDIT BELONGS TO THE PERSON WHO IS ACTUALLY IN THE ARENA; WHOSE FACE IS MARRED BY DUST AND SWEAT AND BLOOD, WHO STRIVES VALIANTLY; WHO ERRS AND COMES SHORT AGAIN AND AGAIN, BECAUSE THERE IS NO EFFORT WITHOUT ERROR AND SHORTCOMING; WHO DOES ACTUALLY STRIVE TO DO DEEDS; WHO KNOWS THE GREAT ENTHUSIASMS, THE GREAT DEVOTION, SPENDS ONESELF IN A WORTHY CAUSE; WHO AT THE BEST KNOWS IN THE END THE TRIUMPH OF HIGH ACHIEVEMENT; AND WHO AT WORST, IF HE OR SHE FAILS, AT LEAST FAILS WHILE DARING GREATLY.

FAR BETTER IT IS TO DARE MIGHTY THINGS, TO WIN GLORIOUS TRIUMPHS EVEN THOUGH CHECKERED BY FAILURE, THAN TO RANK WITH THOSE TIMID SPIRITS WHO NEITHER ENJOY NOR SUFFER MUCH BECAUSE THEY LIVE IN THE GRAY TWILIGHT THAT KNOWS NEITHER VICTORY NOR DEFEAT.

CHAPTER 29

Don't let your ego kill you
Pride and going to the hospital

I remember, as a child, I could do anything physical and not get hurt. All little boys thought that, and some still think that all the way into manhood. I honestly felt I could jump off roofs, fly and land safely without even getting a scratch on me. I knew, beyond a shadow of a doubt, that I was invincible, no matter how lame-brained the stunt of the moment was. As a young man growing up, I thought that was the norm. Of course, when I was a young man, TV shows like Superman, the Green Hornet, and the original Batman series were all over the black and white televisions of America. This invincibility was really my male ego not allowing me to even consider getting hurt. Heaven forbid, that my other friends would find out that I was even slightly concerned with such thoughts.

As a father and grandfather, I now watch the youth of today skateboard down long and winding streets, skirting traffic, jumping over sidewalk rails (let alone skating down the top of those rails to the cement below)...to fall face first into the concrete. Thank goodness that not one of the young men that I have seen pull these stunts, or ones like it, have been hurt in front of me. What makes me shudder is that they, too, think they are invincible. Their egos won't allow them to consider, even for a moment, that their actions could get them into major trouble, and even lead to death. The pride they have in their "ability", driven by massive amounts of youthful testosterone, and Herculean machismo, to them, is a rite of passage into manhood, and a shield against harm and destruction.

Growing up should teach us to be more aware of our abilities, and limitations, as human beings. Unfortunately, some males learn this lesson the easy way, and others (like me) need to be kicked in the head to get my attention and drive the point home. I am sorry, and sad to say, that my lesson almost killed me. I don't want that to happen to you.

As I look back on the heart attack, and those events that lead up to it, I now recognize some of the telltale signs that appeared to me...telling of my impending catastrophe if I didn't change my ways. I didn't recognize the signs, at the time, and my male ego would not let me accept what was about to happen, and the consequences that followed.

BAM! I was stretched out on a cold metal hospital gurney at the brink of death. Why?? I let my ego get in the way of common sense and it almost killed me.

The signs of pending disaster came at me from all directions, but I failed to see them. I was irritable, and easy to anger for no apparent reason. I was out of control financially, due to bad money management, and I had unresolved issues stemming from a previous divorce, left unchecked for years, which I have to take a healthy

If you advance confidently in the direction of your dreams and endeavor to live the life that you have imagined... you will meet with a success unexpected in common hours.
— Henry David Thoreau —

amount of responsibility for, which manifested itself in physical and emotional stress. I am happy to say that I have resolved the past issues, and my Ex and I are on speaking terms again.

And then there were the physical signs that something was terribly wrong, if I had just stopped, backed away, and seen them for what they really were...a heart attack in the making. I remember being very short of breath a lot of the time, mostly from walking very short distances or climbing just a few steps at a time. A day before the incident, I developed a sharp pain in my chest, and a numbness in my left arm...but shrugged it off at the time, and was back to normal (I thought) in short order. I remember thinking it probably was the result of carrying too much of whatever it was I was carrying, or indigestion from the big meal from the day before, and my ego and pride accepted that answer as truth.

As the saying goes, "If I knew then, what I know now" I would have admitted myself into the emergency room at the nearest hospital, instead of letting my EGO control my behavior. I think we men have a major problem with EGO, and issues of this nature, handled by a woman, would be dealt with very differently. Women would recognize that there is something wrong, ask for help from a close family member, or friend, and take care of the problem before it had a chance to fester into something that could possibly not be repaired.

Men, don't let your male ego and pride kill you, like mine almost did. If you feel the signs of heart disease creeping up on you again, like an out-of-control train,

A good scare is worth more to a man than advice.
At this point, we'll downgrade to advice
- Edgar Watson Howe -

swallow your pride, let your ego go, and take care of the problem. If you can't do it for yourself, do it for your family, friends, kids, grandkids, and loved ones. Even if you do the right thing for the wrong reason, you will at least be alive to learn from it the next time. In this instance, you might not have a second chance to make a good impression.

❤ ❤ ❤

He has not learned the first lesson of life who does not every day surmount a fear
- Ralph Waldo Emerson -

CHAPTER 30

Don't be a slave to your credit cards

How many credit cards do you have? I have two. The reality is that it makes absolutely no difference how many credit cards you or I have...if WE control their use, and not the other way around. When I was a younger man, I was terribly in debt. I had allowed my business to fail to the point of having to work three jobs for over two years to get out from under the awful stress it put me in. I used my credit cards for buying food, just so I could eat. The sad part of the whole thing was that a month after I used the card to buy food, I had no idea what I'd spent my money on. Being completely out of control of my financial affairs almost destroyed any semblance of having a normal life. At one point, I spent all the money I had saved, and then proceeded to take my wife on a cruise to the Mexican Riviera using only my credit cards to cover all the expenses with no way to pay them off. Boy, was I out of control.

This bad use of credit cards forced my marriage into a tailspin that I could hardly pull out of. When I married my wife, I observed that she had only one credit card, used it sparingly, and had total control of her finances. She had zero stress, and I was under enormous stress, and all because I fell victim to credit card debt. Besides having to pay off the mountains of interest that accrued from the misuse of the cards, this mis-management of my finances eroded my credibility with my family, kept me away from them for long periods of time while I worked multiple jobs to pay off the loans, and put tremendous strain on my heart. All this happened just after we had gotten married, and six months later I had my heart attack. Was there a correlation between me being out of control of my finances (including credit cards), and my stint in the hospital? Probably. Did I learn from my mishandling of my financials affairs and recover from the tailspin? You bet I did; with a vengeance.

Standing in the kitchen one day, I clearly remember my wife Beth, telling me that the money I earn is not mine, if I owe ANYONE for past purchases. The light finally came on in my head that I couldn't be truly free until I paid off my obligations to those I borrowed from. If you are under mountains of credit card debt, or in debt by any other means, I have been where you are now, and it's not a good place to be.

Years after the fine men and women came back from the Viet Nam war, a lot of them developed what was eventually titled Post-traumatic stress disorder (PTSD). Some veterans still suffer from this today...and have flashbacks confusing past events with present ones. These folks developed all forms of diseases because of the atrocities they witnessed, and lived through over in Viet Nam. The stress related symptoms didn't happen overnight...but sat dormant for months and/or years before they became active and wreaked havoc on these soldiers' bodies, minds, and souls.

I propose that what I developed was what I have coined "Delayed Credit Card Debt Syndrome" (DCCDS™).

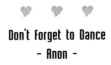

Don't Forget to Dance
- Anon -

Besides the immediate problem of having more money going out of my pocket than I had the ability to pay, the negative symptoms started to pop up over the weeks, and months, after the original bill was past due. I used to get creditors calling at all hours of the day and night to demand payment owed, (which they were certainly entitled to), resulting in more stress laid upon me. I felt guilty that I had gotten myself into such a predicament. My male EGO wouldn't allow me to admit I had made a major mistake.   I became angry at the world, and everyone around me. It affected my job and my attitude. As stated above, the stress it placed on my relationship with my family was extreme. The deeper in debt I got, the more things went wrong. It was a never-ending cycle.

Did I pull out of the nosedive? Yes. Did I learn my lessons about the devastation of not having control of my credit cards and the impact of my actions (or lack of) on my family around me? Absolutely. I now only have two credit cards, which, for the most part, never get used except for emergencies. I guess I am what you would call a survivor of DCCDS(tm) and proud of it. Here's what I learned.

Steps to getting out of credit card debt Hell

 * Pay off the high percentage credit cards FIRST. Reality says that if you have a credit card with 18 percent interest due on the unpaid balance, and another credit card that has a 5 percent interest due on the unpaid balance, you are being charged more interest on the 18 percent card than you

💜   💜   💜

Add each day something to fortify you against poverty and death
- Marcus Annaeus Seneca -

are on the 5 percent credit card. Once you've paid off the higher-interest card, add the monthly amount you would have been paying to the higher-interest card to paying off the lower-interest card, and before you know it, you're credit card debt-free. Or, you may be able to consolidate the 18 percent credit card debt on your 5 percent card. Whatever you can save on interest works in your favor. Remember that these large financial institutions were built on the interest they are charging you each month. They don't make a dime on the amount you've charged on the card, so it's to their benefit to make sure you pay them high interest, month after month, to keep their doors open.

* Also, if you receive a raise, or some other money comes your way, since you're living without that amount already, use those funds to pay down credit card and other debts. Just pretend you never received it, and keep funneling it toward any debt you may have. Once you're debt-free, any money you earn is all yours, to do with as you wish, and that's a great feeling.

* Credit card debt is NOT deductible on your taxes. If you own your own home, look into getting a home equity loan, which usually IS deductible.

* Transfer your credit cards from the high percentage cards to a lower percentage credit card. By doing so, you instantly save the difference between what you are paying and the new

If you do what you have always done,
You'll get what you have always gotten
- Unknown -

percentage. With interest rates being the lowest in many years, it's stupid to have cards with high interest.

* Cut up all but two credit cards. Make these two cards the lowest interest rate cards on the market. Shop around. Having more than two cards is asking for trouble. In this day and age, having a credit card is necessary if you travel, or for emergency services.

* Don't be what credit card companies call a "revolver." Revolvers pay only the minimum amount due every month. You will never get out of debt if you pay off only the minimum.

* Don't EVER be late on a payment. EVER. Two reasons: Once you are late, your credit history is toast. If you're late on a payment, the credit card company does what the industry calls "tiering." It works this way: The first time you are late on a payment, you are hit with a late payment. Now that they have added the late payment to your bill, you have a larger balance due and your minimum amount next month has gone up. Lastly, if you are late on a payment, your credit card company can, and most likely will, increase your interest rate because you are now considered a bad risk.

* The money in your savings account is NOT yours until you pay off your debts - including credit cards. If you have a savings account and say you are getting a whopping 3 1/2 percent on your money, and your credit card debt is 18 percent, you are LOSING 14 1/2 percent on your money every month by having your money in savings. Pay off the credit card debt and realize an immediate 18 percent increase.

There is a universal law of Physics that states: For every action, there is an equal and opposite reaction. If you are in credit card hell, the reaction could be ugly. You are not truly free if you owe debt to the credit card companies. Please, for the sake of you and your family, don't be a slave to your credit card.

❤   ❤   ❤

Money frees you from doing things you dislike.
Since I dislike doing nearly everything, money is handy
- Groucho Marx -

CHAPTER 31

Stress Tips and tricks for successful living

Sometimes the best advice comes from people like you and me. Theory and conjecture is one thing, but sometimes the best cures are the ones that "plain folks" have passed down through the ages based on real world experiences. People that have faced catastrophic calamities to come out the other end with a better sense of what happened, learning from that event, and then taking away survival tips and tricks to help them cope to go on to live a life full to capacity is what it's all about. There are others that may know of little secrets for dealing with the everyday events - that shape our lives. Below is a gathering of ideas and comments - from people, just like you and me, who wanted to share with you some home-grown solutions.

♥

Hmmmm, how do I deal with the stresses of life?

Well, I have to say the best stress-reliever for me is to take a bunch of quarters and go play video poker. I find that my heart rate lessens, and I'm so focused on the cards being dealt (and what my next move should be) that I become very, very relaxed. Even if I'm not winning, the very idea of watching cards flash before me works as a great stress-reducer. I think I actually "zone out" for awhile, becoming completely oblivious to the world around me, which allows me to literally stop, for those minutes or hours, and spend time with me, something I don't often get to do.

Beth Henson, Wife Extraordinaire, Camarillo, CA

My stress management rules changed after my heart attack.... Before it was "don't take life too seriously but do take life problems seriously. "Now I am much less stressed and happier in general to just reverse that to: "don't take life's problems too seriously but do take life seriously... and relish every day." And above all...find something to laugh at each and every day till your side hurts. Important to highlight 'side' here and not 'chest'. Ha.

Chuck Daly, Eagle Rock, CA

I probably have more on my plate than most people I know. I'm married with three young children (8,4 and 2), two dogs and two cats. My father-in-law moved in with us five months ago. I am the main breadwinner for my family - I have a full-time job and direct the LA chapter of a national organization as a volunteer job.

Now with all this, how do I stay sane?

1) I make time for Dianne. I do Pilates followed by Yoga from 7 am - 9:30 am on Sundays. I try to

walk during lunch, even if it's just for a few minutes. 2) Other times I blend family time and exercise. We go to the beach and I go for a walk. We go to the park with the kids on bicycles. I take the dogs for a walk. 3) My mantra is "Delegate and Dump." I try to delegate as much as possible in both my personal and professional lives. I'm not afraid to hire people to help me. I have an assistant at work that backs me up and I have a housekeeper at home. I "buy time" for me by occasionally using the services of a Professional Organizer. She helps me stay on top of the home clutter which I don't have time to deal with during the week, plus she helps me stay up to date with my photo albums. If I can't delegate it, then I try to dump it. Do I personally need to do "it" - whatever it is? 4) I don't let clutter drive me crazy. I used to go nuts with piles. The volume in my life is so high right now that inevitably piles build, which I can't get to. I just don't look at it anymore. 5) I count my blessings. 6) I make time, even if it's just before bed, to visualize and picture things "better and better."

Dianne Gubin, September 13, 2001

❤ ❤ ❤

Those who have easy, cheerful attitudes tend to be happier
than those with less pleasant temperaments regardless
of money, "making it" or success.
- Dr. Joyce Brothers -

♥

I deal with stress by immersing myself in whatever has activated the stress or stress-related action. For example, when the tragedy of September 11, 2001 occurred I watched and read every piece that was available even if I had seen or read it before. By constantly bombarding myself with the information I find it helps me to overcome the issues related to it.

(He is referring to September 11, 2001, the day that terrorists attacked American soil in New York and Washington, D.C.)

Keith Stracke, San Francisco, California

♥

Although I did not have a heart attack—I did go through infertility and it forced me to reevaluate/think about almost every aspect of my life, so I feel that I can relate to a heart attack patient. I am also totally "type a."

Stress handling mechanisms:

Get a massage once a week or every other week. If you cannot get a massage, teach your partner to give you a massage. Become in touch with your body and learn exactly where you hold stress and practice tensing and then relaxing that area. For example, if you hold stress in your shoulders, tense them and let them relax and fall. Also wiggle your toes in your shoes and tense them and let them go—take care of the upper and lower parts of your body!

Yoga—stretching and deep breathing does wonders to get out tension. Yoga forces the body to relax. If you cannot do yoga, a personal trainer can help you with exercises that will help stretch and eliminate tension in problem areas.

Learn to breathe correctly—deep breathing. When you become upset or tense, take several deep breaths until you feel calmer.

Anger—write letters to the person whom you are angry with—vent your anger. Keep a daily journal of your frustrations and also record what made you feel good, so you have some positive things to also write about. Do not be afraid to "praise yourself."

Buy relaxation tapes that teach you how to breathe and release tension from your body. Start with tensing and relaxing the feet and work all the way up to the head, letting go of anger.

Listen to a relaxing CD—maybe one that has the ocean, mountains or woods in the background. If you live near any of these, make sure to take walks as much as possible in tranquil surroundings.

Give yourself breaks during the day—go outside and walk at lunchtime, listen to the birds sing, find a lake, or even a courtyard garden in the city where you have time to think about something else other than work

Join a support group for what is illness you are struggling with and meet others that have been through what you have been through—do not stay in a support group too long, or it becomes a "crutch" and encourages you not to move on—do not dwell on your illness, accept, deal with it, and move on.

Talk about your frustrations—do not keep them inside. Deal with them as they come along—rather than letting them "fester and get worse."

Allow yourself to make mistakes—do not be afraid to let go of "controlling" something, even though it may not be perfect.

Try acupuncture—to unblock blocked energy in the body. Acupuncture forces the body to relax and let go.

Practice letting the mind become "blank" and think about absolutely nothing. This forces both the mind and body to relax

Nurture the spiritual side—whether through "formal religion", prayers, or meditation. Seek healing for anger or whatever is bothering you through prayer and have others promote healing touch and pray for you.

Identify what the stressors are for you and seek to eliminate them in your life. If you hate your job—seek another, if you hate to drive, do not do it. If you are practicing "stress relief" by doing yoga, massage, etc. and you are still totally stressed, change your life to eliminate the "major stressors." Do not wait until you become "ill" to make the changes!

Eat highly nutritious foods, particularly those high in B vitamins. When the body is stressed it burns more B vitamins. Do not seek solace in junk foods, as this will only make the body feel worse. Learn what foods that are nutritious that you really enjoy and make you feel good and concentrate on eating those. Eating nutritionally will help to combat the stress and will also help the body to repair itself. Meet with a nutritionist or personal trainer to figure out a diet that will work for you.

If a person is making you mad—confront that person, let them know what is bothering you and move on. Try and forgive that person. If that is not possible, perhaps you should not have a relationship with that person.

The 12 step program promoted by alcoholics anonymous has quite a few steps about dealing with anger that apply not only to alcoholics, but others as well.

Do not be afraid to ask for help when you need it. If you commit to something and can not get it done, let someone know and do not try and be "Superwoman or superman" and get everything done

Learn to say no when you already have enough to do.

Learn Biofeedback training. Check with your doctor for the location nearest you.

Give yourself some "alone time" everyday, where you are not committed to anything. Use this time to relax or do something that is totally for you

Go to a spa for the day—have a pedicure, manicure, massage, facial, etc. or just hang out in the hot tub, Jacuzzi, pool, etc.

Take a long weekend or vacation and do something that you enjoy—get away from the environment that may be causing you stress—do it for a long enough time period—ideally for at least a week.

For family stress—do not try and change your family—accept the good and bad things about your family and concentrate on what is good. If you do not get along with your family, do accept that and seek a "family" relationship elsewhere—church, friends, club for hobbies, etc. where you enjoy spending time. You do not need to cut your family off, just have realistic expectations and if the relationship is unhealthy, decide what amount of time you are willing to spend.

Research and find out as much as possible about your illness—keep up on new developments. This gives you some semblance of control, when you feel that you have lost control. Do not, however become obsessed and read everything—overly concentrating on your illness is as bad as ignoring it!

Pick a good friend who you can speak frankly with and who can offer you candid advices to help solve problems that are frustrating you.

If you feel that your life is out of control and you are very angry all of the time, seek counseling from a professional to help with anger management.

Kiss your dog. Pets are a great comfort—proven to reduce blood pressure. They always love you and hate to see you upset! Go and pet the dog or bring the cat to sit in you lap and purr away! My dog gives me a kiss when he knows that I am upset and I always feel better!

Ellen Walsh, Port Hueneme, California

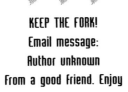

KEEP THE FORK!
Email message:
Author unknown
From a good friend. Enjoy

THERE WAS A WOMAN WHO HAD BEEN DIAGNOSED WITH A TERMINAL ILLNESS AND HAD BEEN GIVEN THREE MONTHS TO LIVE. SO AS SHE WAS GETTING HER THINGS "IN ORDER," SHE CONTACTED HER PASTOR AND HAD HIM COME TO HER HOUSE TO DISCUSS CERTAIN ASPECTS OF HER FINAL WISHES. SHE TOLD HIM WHICH SONGS SHE WANTED SUNG AT THE SERVICE, WHAT SCRIPTURES SHE WOULD LIKE READ, AND WHAT OUTFIT SHE WANTED TO BE BURIED IN. THE

WOMAN ALSO REQUESTED TO BE BURIED WITH HER FAVOR-
ITE BIBLE.

EVERYTHING WAS IN ORDER AND THE PASTOR WAS PRE-
PARING TO LEAVE WHEN THE WOMAN SUDDENLY REMEM-
BERED SOMETHING VERY IMPORTANT TO HER. "THERE'S
ONE MORE THING," SHE SAID EXCITEDLY. "WHAT'S THAT?"
CAME THE PASTOR'S REPLY.

"THIS IS VERY IMPORTANT," THE WOMAN CONTINUED. "I
WANT TO BE BURIED WITH A FORK IN MY RIGHT HAND."
THE PASTOR STOOD LOOKING AT THE WOMAN, NOT KNOW-
ING QUITE WHAT TO SAY. "THAT SURPRISES YOU, DOESN'T
IT?" THE WOMAN ASKED.

"WELL, TO BE HONEST, I'M PUZZLED BY THE REQUEST,"
SAID THE PASTOR.

THE WOMAN EXPLAINED. "IN ALL MY YEARS OF ATTEND-
ING CHURCH SOCIALS AND POTLUCK DINNERS, I ALWAYS
REMEMBER THAT WHEN THE DISHES OF THE MAIN COURSE
WERE BEING CLEARED, SOMEONE WOULD INEVITABLY LEAN
OVER AND SAY, 'KEEP YOUR FORK.' IT WAS MY FAVORITE
PART BECAUSE I KNEW THAT SOMETHING BETTER WAS
COMING...LIKE VELVETY CHOCOLATE CAKE OR DEEP-DISH
APPLE PIE."

"SOMETHING WONDERFUL, AND WITH SUBSTANCE! SO,
I JUST WANT PEOPLE TO SEE ME THERE IN THAT CASKET
WITH A FORK IN MY HAND AND I WANT THEM TO WONDER:
'WHAT'S WITH THE FORK?' THEN I WANT YOU TO TELL
THEM: 'KEEP YOUR FORK...THE BEST IS YET TO COME.'"

THE PASTOR'S EYES WELLED UP WITH TEARS OF JOY AS
HE HUGGED THE WOMAN GOOD-BYE. HE KNEW THIS WOULD
BE ONE OF THE LAST TIMES HE WOULD SEE HER BEFORE
HER DEATH. BUT HE KNEW ALSO THAT THE WOMAN HAD
A BETTER GRASP OF HEAVEN THAN HE DID. SHE KNEW
THAT SOMETHING BETTER WAS COMING.

AT THE FUNERAL PEOPLE WERE WALKING BY THE
WOMAN'S CASKET AND THEY SAW THE PRETTY DRESS SHE

WAS WEARING, AND HER FAVORITE BIBLE, AND THE FORK PLACED IN HER RIGHT HAND. OVER AND OVER, THE PASTOR HEARD THE QUESTION, "WHAT'S WITH THE FORK?" AND OVER AND OVER HE SMILED.

DURING HIS MESSAGE, THE PASTOR TOLD THE PEOPLE OF THE CONVERSATION HE HAD WITH THE WOMAN SHORTLY BEFORE SHE DIED. HE ALSO TOLD THEM ABOUT THE FORK AND ABOUT WHAT IT SYMBOLIZED TO HER. THE PASTOR TOLD THE PEOPLE HOW HE COULD NOT STOP THINKING ABOUT THE FORK AND TOLD THEM THAT THEY PROBABLY WOULD NOT BE ABLE TO STOP THINKING ABOUT IT EITHER. HE WAS RIGHT.

SO THE NEXT TIME YOU REACH DOWN FOR YOUR FORK, LET IT REMIND YOU EVER SO GENTLY, THAT THE BEST IS YET TO COME. FRIENDS ARE A VERY RARE JEWEL, INDEED. THEY MAKE YOU SMILE AND ENCOURAGE YOU TO SUCCEED. THEY LEND AN EAR, THEY SHARE A WORD OF PRAISE, AND THEY ALWAYS WANT TO OPEN THEIR HEARTS TO US. SHOW YOUR FRIENDS HOW MUCH YOU CARE.

AND KEEP YOUR FORK!

CHAPTER 32

Men - Ask for directions

The older I get, the more I realize that men and women are totally different types of people. Not just from a physical standpoint, but from a mental viewpoint. I am not a psychologist by any stretch of the imagination, but I am a keen observer of human nature. My wife and I have seven granddaughters and three grandsons who range from two years of age to the early 20's. Even at the earliest age, the girls ACT differently than the boys...without exception. All the kids live in disparate areas of the west coast, from San Diego, to Seattle, and sorry to say, don't see each other that often so as to observe and emulate each others' behavior.

I guess I am talking about the phenomenon called nature versus nurture. This conversation has been going on for centuries and probably will be discussed in households, university classrooms and in open forums from now to eternity with no absoluteness. But the fact of the matter is, we men see things very differently than women do, particularly when it comes to asking for help, or directions. It may be our male reptilian nature that interferes with our ability to ask for help when help is really needed.

I have been known to drive around in circles for hours looking for a store "that I was sure was RIGHT OVER

THERE" just last week...instead of turning to my wife and consummate travel guide to ask her where that store went. Some of our best arguments are on this subject, and I suspect, if the truth be known, it is true with you, too.

Back to the grandkids. After doing enormous amounts of research on this topic I have concluded that girls, starting from the earliest age, ask for help and assistance when they run into a problem that needs to be solved. Little boys on the other hand (for the most part) want to "do it themselves" no matter how long it takes. As girls get older, they seem to be more attuned to asking for assistance, getting advice from anywhere and anybody that has the knowledge they need to solve a problem and then solve the problem before it festers and gets bigger than it really is. We men (myself included) absolutely refuse (until my heart problem) to ask for help from anyone...even though I knew... "they" knew.

Men - ASK for directions. Take the easy way out. Swallow the ego, cut your losses, swallow the pride, turn to your spouse, friend, lover, or whomever is sitting next to you (who's female) in the car seat...you know, the one just to the right of you, and ASK for directions. Or stop at a gas station in the area. It's one of the easiest things for me to do in my life now that I have learned how. The act of asking for directions has most undoubtedly removed large amounts of stress from my life...and saved me from myself in ways I can't imagine.

If you are a woman - teach your significant other that it's OK to ask for directions. Show us that our egos won't be bruised beyond repair with this newfound knowledge and power. Teach us and we will be beholding to you for all eternity, and the benefit of this is that we may be better to live with AND get to our destination that much faster. The joy of it all.

❤   ❤   ❤

"BASEBALL HEROES"
Contributed via the Internet
By Rabbi Paysach Krohn

IN THE COMPETITIVE WORLD OF THE 1990S, ONE WON-
DERS WHETHER THE OLD ADAGE STILL HOLDS TRUE: "IT'S
NOT WHETHER YOU WIN OR LOSE, BUT HOW YOU PLAY THE
GAME."

THE FOLLOWING TRUE STORY ILLUSTRATES THE POWER OF
HUMAN CONCERN - EVEN IN THE FACE OF INTENSE COMPETI-
TION.

IN BROOKLYN, NEW YORK, CHUSH IS A SCHOOL THAT
CATERS TO LEARNING-DISABLED CHILDREN. SOME CHILDREN
REMAIN IN CHUSH FOR THEIR ENTIRE SCHOOL CAREERS,
WHILE OTHERS CAN BE MAINSTREAMED INTO CONVENTIONAL
JEWISH SCHOOLS. THERE ARE A FEW CHILDREN WHO AT-
TEND CHUSH FOR MOST OF THE WEEK AND GO TO A REGU-
LAR SCHOOL ON SUNDAYS.

AT A CHUSH FUND-RAISING DINNER, THE FATHER OF A
CHUSH CHILD DELIVERED A SPEECH THAT WOULD NEVER BE
FORGOTTEN BY ALL WHO ATTENDED. AFTER EXTOLLING THE
SCHOOL AND ITS DEDICATED STAFF, HE CRIED OUT, "WHERE
IS THE PERFECTION IN MY SON SHAYA?" EVERYTHING THAT
GOD DOES IS DONE WITH PERFECTION. BUT MY CHILD CAN-
NOT UNDERSTAND THINGS AS OTHER CHILDREN DO.

MY CHILD CANNOT REMEMBER FACTS AND FIGURES AS
OTHER CHILDREN DO. WHERE IS GOD'S PERFECTION?"

THE AUDIENCE WAS SHOCKED BY THE QUESTION, PAINED
BY THE FATHER'S ANGUISH, AND STILLED BY HIS PIERCING
QUERY.

"I BELIEVE," THE FATHER ANSWERED, "THAT WHEN GOD
BRINGS A CHILD LIKE THIS INTO THE WORLD, THE PERFEC-
TION THAT HE SEEKS IS IN THE WAY PEOPLE REACT TO
THIS CHILD."

HE THEN TOLD THE FOLLOWING STORY ABOUT HIS SON SHAYA:

SHAYA ATTENDS CHUSH THROUGHOUT THE WEEK AND A BOY'S YESHIVA (TORAH INSTITUTE) ON SUNDAYS. ONE SUNDAY AFTERNOON, SHAYA AND HIS FATHER CAME TO THE YESHIVA AS HIS CLASSMATES WERE PLAYING BASEBALL. THE GAME WAS IN PROGRESS AND AS SHAYA AND HIS FATHER MADE THEIR WAY TOWARDS THE BALLFIELD, SHAYA SAID, "DO YOU THINK YOU COULD GET ME INTO THE GAME?"

SHAYA'S FATHER KNEW HIS SON WAS NOT AT ALL ATHLETIC, AND THAT MOST BOYS WOULD NOT WANT HIM ON THEIR TEAM. BUT SHAYA'S FATHER UNDERSTOOD THAT IF HIS SON WAS CHOSEN IN, IT WOULD GIVE HIM A COMFORTABLE SENSE OF BELONGING.

SHAYA'S FATHER APPROACHED ONE OF THE BOYS IN THE FIELD AND ASKED, "DO YOU THINK MY SHAYA COULD GET INTO THE GAME?"

THE BOY LOOKED AROUND FOR GUIDANCE FROM HIS TEAMMATES. GETTING NONE, HE TOOK MATTERS INTO HIS OWN HANDS AND SAID, "WE ARE LOSING BY SIX RUNS AND THE GAME IS ALREADY IN THE EIGHTH INNING. I GUESS HE CAN BE ON OUR TEAM AND WE'LL TRY TO PUT HIM UP TO BAT IN THE NINTH INNING."

SHAYA'S FATHER WAS ECSTATIC AS SHAYA SMILED BROADLY. SHAYA WAS TOLD TO PUT ON A GLOVE AND GO OUT TO PLAY SHORT CENTER FIELD.

IN THE BOTTOM OF THE EIGHTH INNING, SHAYA'S TEAM SCORED A FEW RUNS BUT WAS STILL BEHIND BY THREE. IN THE BOTTOM OF THE NINTH INNING, SHAYA'S TEAM SCORED AGAIN - AND NOW WITH TWO OUTS AND THE BASES LOADED AND THE POTENTIAL WINNING RUNS ON BASE, SHAYA WAS SCHEDULED TO BE UP. WOULD THE TEAM ACTUALLY LET SHAYA BAT AT THIS JUNCTURE AND GIVE AWAY THEIR CHANCE TO WIN THE GAME?

SURPRISINGLY, SHAYA WAS TOLD TO TAKE A BAT AND TRY TO GET A HIT. EVERYONE KNEW THAT IT WAS ALL BUT

IMPOSSIBLE, FOR SHAYA DIDN'T EVEN KNOW HOW TO HOLD THE BAT PROPERLY, LET ALONE HIT WITH IT. HOWEVER AS SHAYA STEPPED UP TO THE PLATE, THE PITCHER MOVED IN A FEW STEPS TO LOB THE BALL IN SOFTLY SO SHAYA SHOULD AT LEAST BE ABLE TO MAKE CONTACT.

THE FIRST PITCH CAME IN AND SHAYA SWUNG CLUMSILY AND MISSED. ONE OF SHAYA'S TEAMMATES CAME UP TO SHAYA AND TOGETHER THEY HELD THE BAT AND FACED THE PITCHER WAITING FOR THE NEXT PITCH. THE PITCHER AGAIN TOOK A FEW STEPS FORWARD TO TOSS THE BALL SOFTLY TOWARDS SHAYA.

AS THE NEXT PITCH CAME IN, SHAYA AND HIS TEAM-MATE SWUNG THE BAT AND TOGETHER THEY HIT A SLOW GROUND BALL TO THE PITCHER. THE PITCHER PICKED UP THE SOFT GROUNDER AND COULD EASILY HAVE THROWN THE BALL TO THE FIRST BASEMAN. SHAYA WOULD HAVE BEEN OUT AND THAT WOULD HAVE ENDED THE GAME.

INSTEAD, THE PITCHER TOOK THE BALL AND THREW IT ON A HIGH ARC TO RIGHT FIELD, FAR AND WIDE BEYOND THE FIRST BASEMAN'S REACH. EVERYONE STARTED YELL-ING, "SHAYA, RUN TO FIRST! SHAYA, RUN TO FIRST!" NEVER IN HIS LIFE HAD SHAYA RUN TO FIRST.

HE SCAMPERED DOWN THE BASELINE WIDE EYED AND STARTLED. BY THE TIME HE REACHED FIRST BASE, THE RIGHT FIELDER HAD THE BALL. HE COULD HAVE THROWN THE BALL TO THE SECOND BASEMAN WHO WOULD TAG OUT SHAYA, WHO WAS STILL RUNNING. BUT THE RIGHTFIELDER UNDERSTOOD WHAT THE PITCHER'S INTENTIONS WERE, SO HE THREW THE BALL HIGH AND FAR OVER THE THIRD BASEMAN'S HEAD, AS EVERYONE YELLED, "SHAYA, RUN TO SECOND! SHAYA, RUN TO SECOND."

SHAYA RAN TOWARDS SECOND BASE AS THE RUNNERS AHEAD OF HIM DELIRIOUSLY CIRCLED THE BASES TOWARDS HOME. AS SHAYA REACHED SECOND BASE, THE OPPOSING SHORTSTOP RAN TOWARDS HIM, TURNED HIM TOWARDS THE

DIRECTION OF THIRD BASE AND SHOUTED, "SHAYA, RUN TO THIRD!"

AS SHAYA ROUNDED THIRD, THE BOYS FROM BOTH TEAMS RAN BEHIND HIM SCREAMING, "SHAYA, RUN HOME! SHAYA, RUN HOME!"

SHAYA RAN HOME, STEPPED ON HOME PLATE AND ALL 18 BOYS LIFTED HIM ON THEIR SHOULDERS AND MADE HIM THE HERO, AS HE HAD JUST HIT THE "GRAND SLAM" AND WON THE GAME FOR HIS TEAM.

"THAT DAY," SAID THE FATHER WHO NOW HAD TEARS ROLLING DOWN HIS FACE, "THOSE 18 BOYS REACHED THEIR LEVEL OF PERFECTION. THEY SHOWED THAT IT IS NOT ONLY THOSE WHO ARE TALENTED THAT SHOULD BE RECOGNIZED, BUT ALSO THOSE WHO HAVE LESS TALENT. THEY TOO ARE HUMAN BEINGS, THEY TOO HAVE FEELINGS AND EMOTIONS, THEY TOO ARE PEOPLE, THEY TOO WANT TO FEEL IMPORTANT."

HAVE A VERY SPECIAL DAY, AS SPECIAL AS EACH OF YOU ARE.

CHAPTER 33

Love and caring is the best medicine in the world

News Flash!! Social isolation is a hindrance to medical recovery in patients with heart disease. Close social ties have been proven to have profound physical and psychological benefits in curing people with heart problems, as well as other chronic illnesses.

A benefit of being loved and cared about, within the family unit or as a member of a support group, provides you with a sense of closeness, self-care, camaraderie, and laughter at a critical time in your life, and to offset the reality of being frustrated, depressed, isolated, physically lonely, and feeling alone with your illness.

The worst thing to do in times of hurting is to clam up. Intimate relationships breed intimate conversations with people who care, and/or have the same illness. This intimacy builds a sense of oneness with no judgment involved, and builds bridges between otherwise strangers, and allows for the development of coping skills.

As an isolationist, we become singularly focused on our problems, and forget about the world around us. This focus inward ADDS to the stress; conversely, being part of a group allows us to have a better perspective on our own problems. This fact alone has been proven to be an enormous stress reducer.

The social environment of a support group (or a loving family, friends, relatives, and spouses) is to have the encouragement to better take care of your physical, and mental, well-being. Members of this group tend to help you through the rough times, by discouraging the development of a pessimistic attitude, and to support the formation of good behavior patterns by assisting you in developing healthy ways of handling anger, depression, anxiety, nutrition, and the implementation of exercise into your daily routine.

Taking responsibility of one's self to talk openly with family, friends, or participating in a social support group greatly extends the care that a physician can provide after you leave the hospital. The reality is - doctors can't take the time to administer a sense of closeness and comfort to all their patients, even though they might have to desire to do so.

As the world becomes more mobile, we all tend to get more isolated from our family, and friends, and travel farther and farther away from the "family farm." Being socially isolated during an illness may be a harbinger for future serious medical calamities. Conversely, surrounding ourselves with close companionship may be like donning a suit of armor before going out into the battlefield. Equally as important as the armor is the surrounding of oneself with the love, compassion, companionship, and healing energy that a support group has to offer.

The physical benefits may entice you to consider not becoming a isolationist. There are a number of studies that have been performed in recent years that document that being socially isolated increased the release of stress hormones (the bad stuff) into the blood stream, thus setting off a number of psychological as well as physiological changes in the body, some of which are: Elevated blood pressure, poor metabolizing of blood sugar, decrease in immune function, and general feelings of anxiety and depression. Having a strong social surrounding filled with love and caring provides an outlet for this built up stress, and decreasing the stress hormones, thus lowering blood pressure, normalizing the immune systems and bringing the blood sugar levels back into normal ranges, allowing the body now to heal and deal more effectively with emotional stress.

Being part of a support group provides its members with a feeling that they are not alone in the universe, and that there is someone else that has walked in their shoes, and can fully understand what they are going through and how they truly feel. This oneness with the larger mosaic legitimizes the experiences and feelings they may be experiencing. What is heard by its members, most likely is "I am not alone", and the participant may finally realize that there is help available - just for the asking.

I was fortunate to have a wonderful family support group to get me through my darkest hours. Are you alone, either by choice or by design? May I suggest you consider the curative power of companionship, and opening yourself up to being loved and cared for in times of physical, or emotional turmoil? Set aside your natural tendency to want to be alone and the feeling that you can handle this sickness by yourself, and know that other people may need to be hearing that they are not alone. By giving and receiving hugs, talking and being talked too, listening and being listened to, and caring for and being cared for, - and giving of yourself to others in need, you may receive far more than you give out, and remember...

Love and caring is the best medicine in the world.

Family life is the source of the greatest human happiness
- Robert J. Havighurst -

CHAPTER 34

Shake it off...and step up
How are you handling your adversity?

There's an old parable that goes something like this. There was an old farmer that owned a very old mule. One day the old wrinkled mule was walking around the farm and inadvertently fell into an open, and very deep pit. What was the mule to do? After quite a long time in the pit, the old mule decided to call out to his master, thinking that the old farmer would hear his cries and come to his rescue. The farmer arrived at the pit, assessed the situation, and decided that it would be more costly and time consuming to rescue the old mule than to call his neighbors over, put the mule out of his misery, bury the old mule, and then go to town the next day, and buy a younger mule.

The neighbors bought the story, and began to fill in the pit, with the plan to cover the old mule - one shovel full of dirt at a time. The old mule was struck with hysteria, and then realized that if he didn't do something, and do it fast, he was a goner.

As the dirt started to fly, he thought of what action he should take to save himself, and survive. The old mule realized that if he were to let the dirt hit his back, he could shake his back, forcing the dirt to fall all around him onto the floor of the pit. He would then step up onto the newly tossed dirt now covering the floor. He figured that he could repeat this series of steps...to shake it off...then step up, one shovel full after shovel full until he was out of the pit and out of danger. As more dirt got tossed into the pit, the pit filled up with dirt, and he got closer to open air and freedom. And that's exactly what he proceeded to do.

To encourage himself, he would mentally say, "Shake it off and step up...shake it off and step up...shake it off and step up." No matter how dirty he got, how distraught he became, or how much panic he was under...he kept on shaking it off and stepping up.

Out of sheer willpower, determination, and keeping his goal firmly in sight, he shook off the last of the dirt and stepped out...into fresh air, and cool green grass. Instead of accepting defeat, and just laying down to die, he developed a new approach to adversity.

How are you handling your adversity? Have you given in to despair, defeat, and giving up...or have you learned to shake it off and step up to life's challenges? Have you had people tell you to just accept your lot in life...and that there is nothing you can do about it? Look around you, and I guarantee you that there are people you know that are like the old mule who would not accept giving into defeat, or despair, but, instead used adversity as a powerful tool, to shake it off and step up to the wonders of the world, and a new way of dealing with life's little problems.

And remember...the next time someone tosses dirt on your back...shake it off and then step up.

🖤 🖤 🖤

The best things in life must come by effort from within, not by gifts from the outside.
- Fred Corson -

♥ ♥ ♥

How I take care of Stress...I make it leave!!!
Contributed by Candy Finn

I SURVIVED A DOUBLE MASTECTOMY THAT I REQUESTED!!! THAT'S RIGHT, I ASKED FOR IT! NO, I DIDN'T HAVE CANCER, TUMORS, OR ANYTHING ELSE THAT REQUIRED THE SURGERY. HAVE I HAD ANY EXPERIENCE WITH STRESS AND CANCER? YOU BET! MY FAMILY HISTORY HAS LEFT ME A LEGACY FULL OF CANCER. TALK ABOUT STRESS-FUL! BETWEEN MY MOTHER AND FATHER, THEY EXPERI-ENCED THROAT CANCER, KIDNEY CANCER, LUNG CANCER, VAGINAL CANCER, BREAST CANCER (TWICE) AND COLON CANCER (TWICE). MY SISTER'S BREAST CANCER CAME TO HER AT THE AGE OF 49! I LOST MY FATHER TO CANCER AT THE YOUNG AGE OF 60 AND I LOST MY MOTHER TO CAN-CER THIS YEAR AT THE AGE OF 73. NEITHER OF THEM WAS READY TO GO…THEY HAD SO MUCH LIFE IN THEM. IT MADE ME THINK…AND THINK…AND THINK.

I DID NOT TAKE THIS DECISION LIGHTLY. I SPOKE TO MY GENERAL PRACTITIONER, SEVERAL ONCOLOGISTS, AND A COUPLE OF PLASTIC SURGEONS. I MULLED OVER THE DE-CISION TO REMOVE BOTH OF MY HEALTHY BREASTS FOR WELL OVER A YEAR. I WAS ONLY 48 YEARS OLD AND HAD BEEN MARRIED ABOUT 5 YEARS. WOULD THIS BE FAIR TO MY HUSBAND? HOW WOULD I FEEL ABOUT MY FEMINISM? HOW MUCH WOULD IT HURT? WHAT WOULD THE RECON-STRUCTION LOOK LIKE? WOULD I BE DEFORMED FROM THAT POINT ON? THE QUESTIONS WERE NUMEROUS, BUT THE ANSWERS WERE ALL SO CLEAR TO ME.

I AM A VERY POSITIVE PERSON! I HANDLE MY STRESS WITH A POSITIVE ATTITUDE AND THE BELIEF THAT EVERY-THING HAPPENS FOR THE BEST! THE DOCTORS TOLD ME THAT I HAD A 95-98 PERCENT CHANCE OF GETTING BREAST

CANCER SOMETIME IN MY FUTURE, BUT THAT WITH THIS SURGERY, MY CHANCES OF GETTING THE CANCER WOULD DROP TO APPROXIMATELY 5 PERCENT. I DON'T KNOW ABOUT YOU, BUT I REALLY LIKED THOSE ODDS. SO I HAD THE SURGERY!

YOU WILL NEVER KNOW THE RELIEF I FEEL EVERY DAY IN NOT LOOKING OVER MY SHOULDER WONDERING JUST WHEN THIS DREADED CANCER WILL HIT ME! I LOVE MY LIFE! I TRY TO LIVE EVERY DAY TO IT'S FULLEST!

MY FATHER TAUGHT ME MANY THINGS, BUT TWO OF THE THINGS HE TAUGHT ME REALLY STAND OUT. THEY ARE:

1. EVERYTHING HAPPENS FOR A REASON (OR FOR THE BEST).

2. EVERY DAY IN EVERY WAY, IF YOU LOOK HARD ENOUGH, YOU WILL FIND HUMOR IN EVERYTHING.

OUR FAMILY LIVED ON HUMOR AND ENJOYED OUR LIVES TOGETHER MUCH MORE THAN IT SEEMED ANY OF OUR NEIGHBORS OR FRIENDS DID. I THANK BOTH OF MY PARENTS FOR INSTILLING THE LOVING, CARING, POSITIVE ATTITUDE I LIVE BY TODAY. THEY WERE THE GREATEST!

ALWAYS REMEMBER: LIVE WELL, LAUGH OFTEN, LOVE MUCH!

CHAPTER 35

Do you have the Disease of "More?"
There is a difference between quality and quantity of life

It's never enough. No matter how much we have...we always want more. If you make $50,000 per year, then you want 60, and then 70, or higher. If you have a VW rabbit, it's not good enough. We want a Corvette, or BMW, or SUV. It's not good enough to go to a local park for a weekend getaway, is it? No. We need to go to Disneyland or Disney World, spending all our hard earned money to go on a blowout vacation. We fight with the crowds, high prices, and long lines...when a quiet walk on the beach holding hands with your loved ones, and/or your kids has more curative powers than any high priced vacation would ever have. Why? Because it's really not enough!!

I call this affliction, the "Disease of More." And for most people, they have no idea they have it.

If we have a little, we want more, if we have a lot, we need to have a lot more, the cycle never ends until we crash and burn.

Do you have this problem, this disease of "More?" Its very easily recognizable if you know the signs. When you get your paycheck, you get upset, because the government took more than you thought they should, even though you have all you need. When you get in your car, and it doesn't have the smell of a new car with that "leather" interior, you get upset, even though you have a perfectly fine automobile that gets you around town, in comfort, with no mechanical problems.

Every waking hour you are consumed by your need of having to have more of whatever you think you are missing.

I used to be that way...and I didn't recognize the signs either, until it was too late. Then I had a heart attack. I was not happy with what I did have. A loving wife (who was and is my best friend), a wonderful home to hang my hat, and great kids, grandkids, parents, and friends. I was restless inside and REALLY needed to have more. At one point, I knew I wanted and needed more...but of what I did not know. This disease of "more" had taken on a life of its own, and it became a monster of enormous negative ramification, to me, and everyone around me.

My need for "stuff" almost consumed me beyond repair. Are you at that level? Are you so driven by success, and all the trappings that come with this success, that you have lost sight of what living is really about? I developed high blood pressure, sweaty palms, an irritable disposition, short temper...and all because I had a severe attack of wanting "more".

It came to me just recently that all that I needed, I already had. I focused on what I had, and how valuable what I had truly was to me. I came to realize that my wife, my kids and grandchildren, my friends, and the air that I breathe...are more precious to me now than all the gold in Fort Knox.

Don't get me wrong. It's great to have goals and dreams. Beth and I have lots of them, and we work together and enjoy the journey toward their fulfillment. But, I am not consumed by a misguided need for always wanting "more". I have learned to recognize the difference. At times, after we look at what we want...we get it knowing full well it truly is just that...a "want" and not a "need". I now KNOW the difference and this knowledge has set me free.

Beth and I have learned to distinguish between what we "need" and what we "want". Food on the table, a warm house, good transportation, our health, and the love our family and friends is a "need". Going to Bermuda on vacation, a BMW, or a 60-foot sailboat, to us, is definitely a "want". Can you tell the difference between what you need and want in your lives? If you could be honest in your self-assessment, you may be surprised at what you discover is truly a need and what is considered a want.

I am not saying to chuck all the toys that you have accumulated over the years from the hard work you have performed. What I am suggesting is that you look at these "toys" objectively for what they really are...and realize that they are just "things". What's important is that you control the disease of "more" and not let it control you. Don't try to keep up with the Joneses, buying bigger and bigger houses just because of this insatiable NEED to have more. I know a lot of people today that are so tied into wanting "More" just because, and not really understanding why they feel that way.

Realize what is truly important to you and your loved ones, and don't get sucked into the disease of "more".

Remember, the future is not guaranteed to anyone. We only have this moment. Today is all we really need, and everything else is extra.
- Brad Henson -

CHAPTER 36

Change your attitude - cure your heart

We've all heard these statements, haven't we? "Your attitude sucks." "You have a bad attitude." "If you don't change your attitude, you are going to be sent to your room." "It's that attitude that always gets you in trouble with the boss."

Having a negative attitude is like a poison that flows through the body and out into the world, coloring how you react to the world, and how it reacts to you. You see that world through angry eyes, distrusting of everyone and everything that comes in contact with you. The smallest irritations set you off, which most likely raises your blood pressure and could be setting you up for a major fall.

A positive attitude has the opposite effect. Everything looks rosy. The sky is blue, the birds are singing, you love everyone, and everyone loves you.

Have you noticed that when you are in a great mood, have a positive and wonderful attitude, that everything is right with the world? It seemed like the seven dwarfs always had a great attitude - singing, "whistle while you work" in the movie "Snow White and the Seven Dwarfs."

I am sure that if those little dwarfs were real people, they would have the lowest possible blood pressure, no disease, and received great promotions and raises on a very regular basis...all because they believed in having and showing a positive attitude.

In his book *How to Win Friends and Influence People*, Mr. Dale Carnegie states "if you want to be enthusiastic, then act enthusiastic." What he is saying is that if you want to have a wonderfully positive attitude, then act like you already have one. The first secret to a positive attitude is acting like you already have one.

What else can we do about correcting bad attitudes and start healing our heart? First, don't hang around people that have bad attitudes. A bad attitude could and will become a comfortable habit if you let it run unchecked in your life and not deal with it. Just like the phrase "love is contagious", - so too is a bad attitude...if you let it be that way.

Surround yourself with loving, caring, positive-attitude people. Stick with winners, not losers. Your family should be the biggest supporter of your recovery plan. You certainly don't want to hear that you will never get better, now do you? - and then start to believe what you are being told. Be around the people who unconditionally love you the most.

If you have a neighbor with a rotten disposition, tell him/her so...and if they don't change, lose them as friends...if they were ones to begin with.

Don't think that having a bad attitude is a normal thing, because it's not. You were not born with it. It is a creation of your making. You were born surrounded by love, caring, and enormous amounts of support.

Attitude is our view of it...either good or bad, and having a bad attitude is a choice you make, and a bad one at that.

So, go off into the world a changed person...singing in the shower, saying "hi" to the neighbors as you exit the front door, greet the mail person with a renewed sense of happiness and start seeing the world... as a freshly developed rainbow. And most importantly, see how the world starts to react to you. Change your attitude - change your heart.

♥   ♥   ♥

We are taught you must blame your father, your sisters, your brothers, the school, the teachers – you can blame anyone, but never blame yourself. It's never our fault. But it's always your fault, because if you want to change, you're the one who has to change. It's as simple as that, isn't it?

– Katharine Hepburn –

Get a cat or a dog
Therapeutic benefit of animal ownership discovered

Do you ever notice that whatever happens in our lives, if we have a pet around us, the problems don't seem so bad? When I was growing up, I had German Shepard dogs around me. Even after I went out on my own, as a young man, one year, a little black cat meandered into my life. My wife, Beth, had a cat named Yoda when we got married, and it was fully understood by all that if anything happened between Beth and me, I was the one that would have to go before the cat did.

I came to love that little cat named Yoda. He would jump on the foot of the bed at night and remain there till morning. We became great friends, and eventually I taught him, by example, how to watch TV. I would lie on the floor, and he would curl up in front of me, head turned just the right way...to see what was on the TV screen. He was particularly fond of the "Lassie" series, and the "America's Funniest Home Video" show where animals were spotlighted. It was a mutual admiration society, having Yoda in our lives. We all benefited from the experience.

But why is having a pet around the house so beneficial? First of all, like my cat Yoda, he offered unconditional love...not only in my time of need, but all of the time, and this form of love is extremely beneficial to your overall health. Pets have a very non-judgmental nature about them, and because of this personality trait, pet owners develop a real bond with their pet. By caring for, and taking care of pets, it offers people something "else" to think about. I know, when I had come home from the hospital after my heart attack, I would lie on the bed, and stroke our cat for hours. He normally was quite elusive, as most cats are, but I believe he sensed the need to be at my side. The very act of stroking the cat most likely lowered my blood pressure and removed any stress I was feeling at the time.

In a current study by Dr. Karen Allen, of the State University of New York at Buffalo, she looked at the most stressful people she could find...stockbrokers. For the study, she examined people that used medication to control or lower blood pressure. She wanted to test high achievers, so she picked only men and women who earned in excess of $200,000 per year. Half of the test group was asked to adopt a dog or cat at the beginning of the test. At the end of the trial, the pet owners registered one-half the stress of those that did not own a dog or cat. The interesting outcome to this test was that a large majority of the people who originally did not have a pet during the trial adopted one the first chance they could.

A Johns Hopkins Medical Center study concluded that 50 out of 53 people who owned pets were alive longer than one year after their first heart attack, while 17 out of 39 of those without the furry friends lasted only one year. Another study at the University of California at Los Angeles showed that 1/3 of all Medicare enrollees who owned pets visited the doctors fewer times than the pet-free group.

In 1980, Erika Friedmann, Ph.D, of the University of Pennsylvania unearthed a direct correlation between men who'd had heart attacks indicating an increased rate of survivorship over those that did not. More of a surprise was that men owning a pet were a better predictor of surviving heart disease than these same men having a spouse.

At the Baker Medical Research Institute in Prahan, Australia, Warwick Anderson, M.D. performed a study where he compared the cholesterol levels of 4,957 pet-free, and 784 pet owners. The cholesterol levels of the pet owners were substantially lower.

Benefits of pet ownership have been shown in case study after case study. The human-pet interaction could be just watching some fish swim around a fish tank, or it might be taking the family dog out for a walk, or watching the cat push a ball of string around the kitchen floor. Whatever the activity you may have with a pet, the act gives you time to get away from problems, reflect on the day's events, concentrate on someone else (in this case your pet), and in turn, lower your blood pressure and become very relaxed in the process.

What are the roles that pet ownership plays in our lives? On purely a physical point, we feel safer with a dog around us, which in turn provides us with less stress. Stroking a cat or a dog gives us the comfort of touch. How many times a day, while you are walking to the store, or at a friends house, do you overhear them talking to their pets? We all open up more easily while talking to a pet.

From a physical activity point of view, pet ownership keeps us more energetic. Cats and dogs need to be bathed, and brushed, on a regular schedule, horses should be ridden, fish tanks should be cleaned, litter boxes should be emptied, and all this takes energy.

My wife says that sitting on the couch, with a cat in her lap, purring loudly...is heaven...and some doctors say that this type of activity can reduce blood pressure as much as some medications can.

If you don't have a pet, please consider getting one...for your health and theirs.

❤   ❤   ❤

A small pet animal is often an excellent companion for the sick
- Florence Nightingale -

CHAPTER 38

Link between Faith and Healing found

Fear imprisons, faith liberates; fear paralyzes, faith empowers; fear
disheartens, faith encourages; fear sickens, faith heals; fear makes
useless, faith makes serviceable.
- Harry Emerson Fosdick -

I am writing this chapter in the aftermath of the worst terrorist attack on American soil (or on any soil, for that matter) during peacetime. The attack occurred September 11th, 2001 when four commercial airliners were hijacked and two of them were forced to fly into the twin World Trade Center towers in New York, one plane slammed into the Pentagon building in Washington D.C, and yet another crash landed in a field in Pennsylvania. As of this writing, the death toll is climbing by the thousands, and the final tally won't be known for days, weeks, or months, if ever.

Americans are resilient, resolute, hardy people...who, when confronted, in the face of disaster, rise to uncommon valor physically and mentally, and do whatever it takes to help their fellow man overcome his or her adversity. Part of this resoluteness is finding an inner strength to go on with life, as they know it.

As the United States and the world attempted to get a handle on the magnitude of this cowardly act of terrorism, the President of the United States indicated Friday, September 14th, 2001 as a day of mourning, and he encouraged everyone to attend a lunchtime religious service in a church, synagogue, Mosque, Temple, or congregation, to try to start the healing process. The leaders of the free world understand that before the healing process can begin, tapping into one's faith, saying a prayer and having conversations with a higher power must commence - to come to grips with the sense of loss, the grief, and mourn for those who have died.

The same feelings can come up when one goes through any kind of catastrophic event or illness.

In his book *Healing Power of Faith: How Belief and Prayer Can Help You Triumph Over Disease*, Dr. Harold Koenig says that faith has given his patients a strong sense of mastery over their lives. When the daily rigors of life - illness, money problems, personal conflicts - threaten the stability of their day-to-day lives, these religious folks dig deep into their reserve of motivation and energy and pull out their inner strength to survive. They use this connection to a higher power to fill the gap between their normal endurance level, and what is required of them to handle the problem they face. Religious people see this as a relationship or partnership with someone that can help them get through their problems with a positive outcome.

Surveys have been conducted that indicate over 96 percent of the population of the United States have a belief in a higher spiritual power. This belief is being tested now, more than ever before. My concern is that there is unresolved "anger" in the world today. People have not been taught how to recognize that anger and focus the anger toward the issue that made them angry in the first place instead of taking it out on anyone that gets in their way...(like the terrorists have done). We need to learn how to diffuse the anger and pain, and replace it with love and compassion. Remember, "anger" is only one letter from "danger."

If we, as a society, do not tap into this spirituality and belief system, and do it quickly, we may see a huge increase in medical problems in the near-to-distant future. What is the relationship between faith and healing? Is there a curative power between faith and healing one's wounds...both physically and/or mentally? Numerous Duke University studies have come to light with groundbreaking facts:

* In over 50 to 80 percent of the most common disorders today, people who have a strong belief and/or expectation that they will get better have a profound positive impact on the rate at which they heal.
* People that regularly attend a church service have substantially fewer deaths from coronary artery disease.
* The same study shows that folks that attend religious gatherings have lower diastolic blood pressure than those that don't.
* One medical study has shown that people that were prayed for before, during and after a medical operation had fewer complications after heart surgery.
* Solid findings show that having a strong belief system and faith makes a positive difference in three profound areas: Prevention of illness, coping with illness, and recovery.
* Folks that attend religious services on a regular basis have a much stronger immune system than those who don't. Lower blood levels of interleukin-6 (IL-6), which increases with chronic stress that is not released, has been proven with

people who attend church on a regular basis. It is important to note that high levels of IL-6 indicates a weak immune system, which then increases the risk of autoimmune disease, and certain cancers.

There are over 200 studies that now show the correlation between religious practices and mental and physical health. What has risen from these reports and studies is that you don't have to have a belief in organized religion to benefit. According to Dr. Herbert Benson, from his book *Timeless Healing*, he defines "belief" as being much broader than belief in God. But how does it work? What are the physical links between faith and healing? According to Dr. Benson, the physical brain manifests activity patterns which remembers sickness, and other patterns which remember when you were well. If, at some point you were ill, and then you said to yourself, "I am getting better and better", and you got well, then your brain activities remembered that as being the truth. Then, in the future, when we get sick, and then "believe" that we will get better, the subconscious mind replays that wellness tape, remembering when we were better, and we get better.

We all know people that are eternal optimists or pessimists. Think about their lives for a moment. The pessimist is more depressed, has more sickness, and a more sour disposition than the optimist does. The optimist (of which I am one) sees the day as the beginning of new life, every thing is rosy, and the glass is full to brimming. It is a proven fact that our sub-conscious mind does not make a distinction between what is real and imagined. To validate this hypothesis, Dr. Steven Causlin, professor of Psychology from Harvard University performed an experiment, whereas he had some people glance at a grid. Within that grid he had placed the capital letter "A". He had them continually stare at the center of the grid and the letter A. They stared, and glared and glanced at it for a long period of time. He then took the grid away and performed a positron emission tomography (PET) scan (which provides a picture of brain activity) on the participants. He noticed that a certain part of the brain lit up, way back in the area of the brain called the occipital cortex.

The doctor then had his experimenters stare at a second grid with no letter A in the middle, for approximately the same length of time and had them "visualize" that there was still the letter A in the middle. He then did yet another PET scan of the brain. The results were exactly the same...meaning that the brain did not differentiate between what was real and what was imaginary.

Studies done with athletes were conducted where a group of athletes were split into two groups. One group was taught techniques in visualization and imagery and the power of "belief". This group sat quietly every day and visualized themselves believing they were getting better, and visualized performing their selected sport to perfection - but were not allowed to physically practice that sport.

The other group was not allowed to practice visualization and imagery techniques, but went about practicing every day in their chosen sport. After a set amount of time, the group that visualized themselves getting better and better performed as well, or better, than the group that never stopped practicing, but did not learn the visualization, imagery, or belief techniques that the first group had learned. Why? Most likely it is because the subconscious brain doesn't know the difference between what is real and what is imagined. Your mind/body connection will assist you in developing a "wellness" and your body will respond.

What then is wellness? Webster's defines it as the quality or state of being in good health. Does this mean that we should forgo all medical advice, doctors, pills, and surgical procedures? Absolutely not! Developing the mind/body connection will enhance your wellness. This connection should be in addition to what the medical community has to offer you, not a replacement.

From all the research that has come out in recent years, having a strong spiritual and religious belief system will allow you to live longer than non-religious or spiritual people - if you take action and practice your beliefs. For those non-religious or spiritual minded individuals out there, if you can't believe in a higher power, then have a belief in "belief". These findings show that having a strong belief system, be it religious or spiritual in nature, may be as important to the healing process as not smoking, or cutting down excess alcohol consumption - in surviving or thriving - and how long you live.

Contributed by Arlys Little, Atascadero, California

While driving to the drug store to take my blood pressure one day, I found myself blacking out at one of the busiest intersections. I quickly prayed, "God, please don't let me crash!" I woke up immediately, and blithely continued on. My blood pressure and pulse was a little high, but not enough to worry about, or so I thought!

What felt like bird-wings fluttering in my chest on and off during that day turned out to be ventricular Tachycardia, which is a very fast heartbeat. This was recorded on a monitor later when I finally went to the emergency room. In fact, bells rang, nurses came running, and pandemonium reigned as my heart-beat went out of control.

An angiogram showed I needed a procedure called ablation, to correct the "short circuiting" of the electrical system in my heart. Having little if any control over what would happen next was pretty scary, to say the least.

But something I found to be true years ago gave me peace. Just as God had answered my prayer to keep me safe at the stop-light, he now gave me peace in knowing that whatever the outcome might be, I could rest and put myself in his hands.

Now, months later, I'm doing well. More importantly, I still place myself in his hands every day, as I take time to thank him for my life. I highly recommend prayer (which is really just talking with God) as the most efficient prescription for reducing feelings of stress and anxiety in one's life.

If you'd like to know more details concerning the positive aspects of prayer, you can contact Arlys through Crow Publishing.

❦   ❦   ❦

Religious faith, indeed, relates to that which is above us, but it must arise from that which is within us.
— Josiah Royce —

CHAPTER 39

Hopefulness lives - Hopelessness kills

Sometimes I sit quietly; staring out the window and hope that the rain doesn't come or wish it would come (if we are in a drought). I hope that all my children and grandchildren grow up to live healthy and happy lives. When we were younger, we all had hopes for the future. We hoped that we would be rich like Norman Rockefeller, as good looking as Clark Gable, as suave and debonair as Errol Flynn, or as good a dancer as Fred Astaire. Some of us realized our dreams.

I *hope* you did.

We do grow up. We go about our day-to-day living, finishing school, getting a job, raising a family, having children, and grandchildren, and settling into a comfortable living. For the most part, we men feel good about the future, and hope that all turns out for the best. We men are doers. Action is our middle name. We are going to make it happen, darn it, no matter what obstacles get in our way. It's inbred into the male DNA gene, isn't it? We are optimistic and have tons of hopes tossed into the mix for good luck.

What about the other group of people out there that have fallen off the "hope wagon" with their body and soul? How does their hopelessness affect their life expectancy and their health? One reason that pessimistic or hopeless people are more prone to premature death is that these folks are not likely to be engaged in healthful lifestyles, such as being involved in exercise programs, good hygiene, eating well, and/or taking medications prescribed by their medical practitioner. It seems that hope-less thinking people have LESS of what optimistically hope-full people have.

Susan Everson, Ph.D., an epidemiologist from the Western Consortium for Public Health in Berkeley, California came up with some startling statistics after interviewing approximately 2,428 middle-aged males about their overall outlook on life. Ranking them - from the low- end, as feeling hopeless, to the high-end as hopeful. Coming back and reviewing the findings 10 years later, she discovered that more common than not, men who had maintained a mental state of hope-lessness died prematurely from either cancer or heart disease. Men who were most hopeless in their outlook toward a positive future had three times the death rate over those who were hopeful.

In another study, Dr. Daniel Mark, of Duke University, surveyed 1,719 men and women just before they were going into the operating room for heart surgery. He wanted to find out how much hope these men and women had for a full recovery and to have a full resumption of their pre heart attack daily routines. A year later, 12 percent of the 1,719 interviewees (the pessimist/hopeless thinkers) died. However, only 5 percent of the hopefully optimistic in the group passed away.

Do you ever just "feel" bad when you are sad, frustrated, or just stressed out? Is there a negative physical impact to the body when under extreme levels of emotions? According to Psychiatrist Elizabeth Gullette, M.D., at Duke University, there is a direct correlation between negative emotions and reduced blood flow to the heart. To prove or test their hypothesis, they attached portable monitors that recorded the blood flow into the heart on

132 patients with heart disease, and monitored these people for 48 hours.

During this timeframe, the participants in the study were given diaries to record their activities...including any and all emotions they were feeling at the time. After gathering up the portable monitors, and analyzing the results, they concluded that frustration, sadness, and the emotions of stress doubled the "likelihood" of substantially decreased blood flow. Their findings indicated that intense negative emotions tripled the risk of reduced blood flow, which can then cause angina...and the onslaught of a heart attack.

Ask the question of yourself "Am I a pessimist, or an optimist?" Then go ask your family and friends the same question. When you are at work, pull your boss, and co-workers aside, and ask them how THEY perceive you - hopeful or hopeless (optimistic or pessimistic). Compare how you think of yourself, and how others perceive you. You might be surprised. Listen to your speech patterns. Are your words filled with hopeful statements? After you wake up in the morning and open your eyes for the first time, how do you see the day? If the first sentence out of your mouth is "Crap, I have to go to work today", then most likely you are a pessimist - and you might want to change your behavior.

Don't forget that your survival from your heart attack was truly a gift, a second chance to make a great impression. Don't squander it by being a pessimist.

♥   ♥   ♥

Cheerfulness is as natural to the heart of man in strong health as color to his cheek; and wherever there is habitual gloom there must be either bad air, unwholesome food, improperly severe labor or erring habits of life.
- John Ruskin -

C H A P T E R 40

You are what you eat
Proper nutrition and your heart health

What is the best nutritional guidance available - to reduce the onslaught of having another heart attack in the months, years, or decades ahead, for people who are Type A personality prone? Pick a letter of the alphabet, and there is a diet attached to it. I am not the first to tell you that there are as many diet plans on the market today as there are stars in the sky. One thing to remember in your search for the right "plan" for your Type A lifestyle is that you didn't develop heart disease overnight by going out and eating an occasional high fat content meal of burgers and fries at the local hamburger stand. The dilemma we are in today is of bad habits gone awry over time.

Like the family car that is taken to the car dealership for a lube and oil change every 3,000 miles to keep it running in tip-top shape, so, too, must we constantly eat the correct types of food on a consistent basis to keep our heart and soul in tip-top shape, and our body functioning in prime condition.

So how do we do that? According to the American Heart Association (AHA) Dietary Guidelines, revised in 2000, and intended for the healthcare professional, the major emphasis is on weight management. In this document, the AHA stresses the importance of what they call "avoidance of excess total energy intake, and a regular pattern of physical activity." My take is "eat less, exercise more." The one thing the AHA stresses is to remember is if you have had a recent heart problem, or are concerned with your heart health, consult your doctor before you go on any diet program.

As far as nutrition goes, they suggest consuming less than 30% of your total daily intake of energy in the form of fat. Limit your intake of dietary saturated fat to less than 10 percent and your consumption of cholesterol to less than 300 mg/d. Recent findings indicate that you would benefit by consuming at least two fish servings per week. Because of the concern that high blood pressure needs to be controlled, the AHA now strongly recommends, based on major medical studies, taking in fruits, vegetables, and low-fat dairy products, in addition to limiting salt intake to less than 6 grams per day. Sugar should be curtailed, as well as excessive alcohol consumption.

The AHA states that eating foods from all the food groups helps to ensure we get all the nutrients our bodies need in correct proportions. They stress taking in fruits and vegetables, fat-free and low-fat dairy products whenever possible, cereal and grains, nuts and legumes, along with fish, poultry and lean meats.

Other than eating right, what else can be done to maintain optimal health? Quick things you can do to take control of your eating habits:

* Keep a diary of what you eat. There is a hospital in the San Fernando Valley, in Southern California, that has a diet program where the only thing they do is meet once per week and read the daily diaries from the preceding week. Without fail, the members that write down what they eat ev-

ery day, lose weight and those that don't - don't.
* Move. Nothing happens until you take action. Sounds simple, but the reality is, we could all move more. If the goal is to burn off more energy than we take in, the only thing we can do is MOVE. What would happen if we increased our activity just 10 percent? WOW.
* Drink more water. Just plain water, with no additives. No fair cheating and adding a little something to it to enhance the flavor. Just plain water. By drinking more water, we flush out the body of toxins.
* Don't lie to yourself. If you can't exercise, then call it for what it is -an off day. When I was running track in high school, we had off-days when we didn't work out. We all knew it, and accepted it for what it was - an off day. So don't lie about your off-days.
* Cut down on your portions. I have found that the portions you serve at home and the ones that restaurants serve ARE NOT the same size. When dining out, my wife and I have started sharing meals - one, because the portions are so big and we don't need all that food, and the side benefit is that we save some money. While dining out at our favorite restaurant one evening, years ago, Beth commented how clever the cook was in the restaurant...to know exactly the amount I needed to be served to get full.

Living a healthy, happy, no-limit lifestyle has to do with Balance. The same is true with what we take into our systems. Over the years, I have watched how my wife deals with food. I have seen her on more than one occasion being in the mood for...say, chocolate chip mint ice cream. She proceeds immediately to the freezer with spoon in hand, opens the top of the ice cream container, and while using the back side of the spoon, she scoops out just a little bit of her favorite ice cream. When asked why she only took a little bit, she turns to me, smiling, and says, "that is all my body needed." She is in total control of her nutritional needs. Food to her is a fuel, like gasoline is to a car. No more, no less. Her body knows how much and what it needs to run at optimal proficiency. This way of eating is being in total balance.

Part of this balance is to exercise often, laugh a lot, love and be loved as much as you can, and surround yourself with the companionship of wonderful people. If you learn to add eating a balanced diet to this equation, you have made it to the pinnacle of success.

Ask yourself if food is a luxury item to you, or high-powered jet fuel to make your human body run better, faster, and farther than it has gone before? Only you can accurately and honestly answer that question. You truly are what you eat. Remember -Like in life, proper nutrition has to do with Balance.

♥   ♥   ♥

If you can't fight, and you can't flee - Flow
- Robert Eliot, Cardiologist -

CHAPTER 41

Taking vitamins may lessen onslaught of heart disease risk

The decree goes out across the heartland of America, for moms to unite in the cause to end all causes - the lament is heard by kids everywhere; "you can't leave the table until you eat all your veggies. Don't you to want to grow up big and strong?" At the time, I thought it was a conspiracy. It's an affront to my manhood. Who me? Eat what? But eat I did. Did it make a difference in how big and strong I grew up by being forced to eat all my veggies? Of course it did. But don't tell mom I liked the different colored items she happily put on the plate every day. If the secret were known, I would have eaten them if she forced me to or not. I happen to love veggies. I am now convinced that she (and mothers the world over) have always known the true secret of vegetables.

In the old days, we got all of our minerals and vitamins from the fruits and vegetables that were grown out in the garden, then brought directly into the house, quickly washed, cleaned, cooked, and placed on our plates. For the most part, the fruits and veggies were freshly harvested the same day we consumed them. Times have changed. Today, we go to the local grocery store, rummage through the vegetable racks, choosing what vegetable or fruit items looks like the healthiest from the bunch in front of us, to then take them home to place in the refrigerator for the following day's (or week's) meals.

So what's all the ruckus about today, from the medical community, the news media, and over the Internet, about taking in the right amount of minerals and vitamins to get us and keep us healthy? We surely get all the minerals and vitamins from the foods we eat. Right? Not exactly, according to Dr. Joel Wallach, M.D., known the world over as the "Vitamin Doctor". On numerous occasions he has lectured about the soil depletion problem in the United States and its negative effects on men and women not getting the proper amounts of vitamins, minerals, and trace minerals into their system to fight off the ravages of time and fight and conquer disease.

According to Dr. Wallach, in the early 1930's, the Senate of the United States, released an "official" public document recognizing that farmers were over-farming the lands of America, and consequently removing the essential minerals and vitamins from the soil - and not adequately replenishing lost vitamins and minerals to the land between growing seasons. And that was way back in the 1930's! Just imagine the condition of the soil 71 years later, if there were not a concerted effort to replenish the minerals, vitamins, and trace minerals to the soil.

Just take the time to look at the labels of some of your favorite foods. Most of the items placed in the foods today are to give the foods back their "normal color", or allow them to maintain a very long shelf life, not vitamins and minerals to give US a longer shelf life. Just for fun, compare how many vitamins, minerals, and trace minerals your cat or dog food has in it to some of the canned foods you consume. Hmm, something to think about.

Have you ever wondered why we are hearing of more cancer, heart disease, and other debilitating illnesses in

I am not afraid of storms, for I am learning how to sail my ship.
- Louisa May Alcott -

the last 70 years than in any other time period in history? Could it be that these diseases are being brought on by a "lack" of the correct amounts of minerals and vitamins in the human body, which allows the body to fight off and prevent these deadly diseases from occurring? Perhaps.

So what vitamins and minerals are essential to lessen the onslaught of heart disease risk? If we don't get the right amount and kinds of vitamins, minerals, and trace minerals from the food we consume, then we must supplement to obtain the benefits.

Folic acid and vitamin's B6 and B12

All humans have an amino acid, called Homocysteine (pronounced homo-SIS-teen) that is normally found in the body. The medical community has recently released numerous studies indicating that individuals with high blood levels of Homocysteine may, and could, be increasing the opportunity of contracting stroke, heart disease, and consequent lower blood flow to the hands and feet. The consensus from the medical community is that having high levels of this amino acid may somehow damage the arteries, causing the blood vessels to be less flexible, and making the blood more apt to clot.

Current thinking shows that the levels of this particular amino acid in the blood stream are negatively and positively affected by the consumption of folic acid, vitamin B6 and B12. The National Heart and Lung Institute states that men and women who take in less than their recommended daily amounts of these three vitamins are susceptible to having higher levels of Homocysteine. So what are these recommendations? According to the National Heart and Lung Institute, an individual should take 400 micrograms of folic acid, 200 milligrams of B6, 6 micrograms of B12.

Results of studies show the following: Researchers and scientists at the University of California, San Francisco, show heart disease rates could be lowered by as much as 13 percent for men, and 8 percent for women over the next 10 or so years if people over the age of 35 took in a daily dose of folic-enhanced grains. What's more important to note, however, is that there would be a reduction of 310,000 heart disease- related deaths if folks with higher amounts of homocysteine ingested daily folic acid and B12 by supplementation - in addition to consuming folic-enhanced grains.

Vitamin E

I am sure that most everyone has heard of the benefits of taking in ample amounts of Vitamin E. In a June, 1995, in a copy of the Journal of the American Medical Association (JAMA), a medical study was published documenting the importance of vitamin E, (an antioxidant) in the fight against heart disease. In the study, men with a pre-existing heart condition, and given at least 100 IU of vitamin E per day showed much fewer cases of coronary artery disease over those that had not been given vitamin E. Even nurses got into the act in another test to validate the benefits of taking in larger amounts of vitamin E. 130,000 nurses were given greater than 100 IU's per day of vitamin E, with a results being a 46% reduction in the episodes of heart attacks in women, and 26% in men.

Magnesium, Potassium, Calcium, and Zinc

Magnesium, Potassium, Calcium, and Zinc have all shown the benefits of controlling high blood pressure. Magnesium, for example, helps reduce irregular heart-

♥   ♥   ♥

He who has help has hope, and he who has hope has everything.
Arab Proverb

beats and heart spasms. The walls of the blood vessels have a stronger structural integrity if the appropriate levels of Copper are taken into the body. Having a Copper deficiency has been tied to weaknesses in the walls of the blood vessels, leading to strokes. An engineer would say that having the proper amount of copper in the system would equate to having solid "structural integrity" for the "I" beams (the main support) of a building. Have you ever had a car radiator hose break? It's usually because the wall of the hose has weakened under constant pressure, and over time...weakens to the point where a soft spot forms, ultimately breaking through in the form of a hole. The same thing happens to the walls of the blood vessels.

CoEnzyme Q10

Dr. Fred Crane, from the University of Wisconsin, discovered the importance of CoEnzyme Q10 way back in 1957. His findings proved the importance of this substance to the function of every cell in the human body, including the heart muscle. Through extensive research, he found that levels of Q10 decline starting at around the 30th birthday for both males and females. As the levels of Q10 decreases, so, too, does the general health of the individual.

Other findings have determined that Q10 is important for the manufacturing of cellular energy. The benefits of Q10 supplementation are many, including improving the condition of congestive heart failure, calming arrhythmia. Q10 acts as a very powerful antioxidant by keeping free radicals at bay, and improves the overall efficiency of the body's immune system and lowers blood pressure.

Selenium

Selenium, another essential vitamin for optimum heart health, protects the body from the ravages of coronary artery disease. Having the correct amounts of Selenium in the body has been proven to ward off the onslaught of arthritis and cancer.

It is common knowledge throughout the medical community that minerals, trace minerals, and vitamins all work together, meaning that they are synergistic. Its like Ying and Yang. Vitamin E is a partner of Selenium. If Magnesium is to work properly, then other vitamins, such as Vitamin E, B Complex, and C must be present in proper amounts. It all has to do with Balance.

Go to your doctor and have him/her test you for vitamins, minerals, and trace mineral deficiency. Do your own research. My belief is that my heart attack could have been completely avoided, if I would have known of the information in this chapter about vitamins, minerals, and trace minerals...in addition to the benefits of modifying my lifestyle by introducing more mental, spiritual, and physical balance to the equation.

♥   ♥   ♥

What Happiness is
Author Unknown

WE CONVINCE OURSELVES THAT LIFE WILL BE BETTER AFTER WE GET MARRIED, HAVE A BABY, THEN ANOTHER. THEN WE ARE FRUSTRATED THAT THE KIDS AREN'T OLD ENOUGH AND WE'LL BE MORE CONTENT WHEN THEY ARE. AFTER THAT WE'RE FRUSTRATED THAT WE HAVE TEENAGERS TO DEAL WITH. WE WILL CERTAINLY BE HAPPY WHEN THEY ARE OUT OF THAT STAGE. WE TELL OURSELVES THAT OUR LIFE WILL BE COMPLETE WHEN OUR SPOUSE GETS HIS OR HER ACT TOGETHER, WHEN WE GET A NICER CAR, ARE ABLE TO GO ON A NICE VACATION, WHEN WE RETIRE.

THE TRUTH IS, THERE'S NO BETTER TIME TO BE HAPPY THAN RIGHT NOW.

IF NOT NOW, WHEN?

Your life will always be filled with challenges. It's best to admit this to yourself and decide to be happy anyway. One of my favorite quotes comes from Alfred D Souza. He said, "For a long time it had seemed to me that life was about to begin - real life. But there was always some obstacle in the way, something to be gotten through first, some unfinished business, time still to be served, a debt to be paid. Then life would begin. At last it dawned on me that these obstacles were my life".

This perspective has helped me to see that there is no way to happiness.

Happiness is the way. So, treasure every moment that you have. And treasure it more because you shared it with someone special, special enough to spend your time and remember that time waits for no one.

So stop waiting until you finish school, until you go back to school, until you lose ten pounds, until you gain ten pounds, until you have kids, until your kids leave the house, until you start work, until you retire, until you get married, until you get divorced, until Friday night, until Sunday morning, until you get a new car or home, until home is paid off, until spring, until summer, until fall, until winter, until you are off welfare, until the first or fifteenth, until your song comes on, until you've had a drink, until you've sobered up, until you die, until you are born again to decide that there is no better time than right now to be happy.

Happiness is a journey, not a destination. Work like you don't need money, Love like you've never been hurt, And dance like no one's watching.

CHAPTER 42

Take an aspirin a day

C an a drug that has been on the market for over a hundred years be useful in reducing the risk of modern day medical calamities such as secondary heart attacks, and strokes? Here comes the disclaimer:

As far back as the 1920's, in advertising campaigns with banners like "Aspirin does not affect the heart", ads were used to dispel the climate at the time that such drugs could damage the heart. In 1999, articles professing, "Aspirin has been found to reduce the risk of death and/or nonfatal myocardial infarction in patients who have previously experienced infarction or unstable angina pectoris" are common.

Aspirin has become so beneficial that some of the largest drug companies that manufacture and market the drug carry the American Heart Association's seal to highlight the cardiovascular effects. One aspirin manufacturer states in its documentation that of the 80 million aspirin tablets that American's consume daily, a large majority are taken for reduction of heart disease symptoms, and not for everyday aches and pains.

Even though the modern day version of "Aspirin", in its current form, was introduced 100 years ago, the history of the drug can be traced back to the time of Hippocrates. His followers were advised to gnaw on the leaves of willow trees, thus alleviating their aches and pains. The Chinese got into the act by using the bark of the same tree to control fevers. Different bark derivatives were analyzed in the early 1800's that would be more easily tolerated by the human body, and acetylsalicylic acid (Aspirin's chemical name) was discovered.

Aspirin works by blocking certain prostaglandin in the body...thus lowering body temperature, relieving inflammation, relieving minor aches, and most importantly, interfering with the role that blood platelets perform in forming clots. Blood clots occur by these platelets grouping together. By using Aspirin, the platelets are made to be less "sticky", and less successful in allowing the platelets to come together as a group to develop into blood clots - not allowing the manufacture of prostaglandins.

Dr. Charles H. Hennekens, M.D, and Dr. P.H. John Snow, Professor of Medicine and Ambulatory Care and Prevention, Harvard Medical School and Chief, Division of Preventative Medicine Brigham and Women's Hospital, stated "The widespread use of aspirin during acute heart attacks would avoid 5,000 premature deaths in the United States alone." A total of 10,000 lives would be saved if aspirin were more widely used for prevention of second heart attacks and at the onset of symptoms of a first heart attack."

There are just too many studies to quote them all, so PLEASE, do your own research and see for yourself the benefits of taking a daily regiment of aspirin. It may save your life, or that of a loved one near you.

Since the use of aspirin is not without some risk in some people, you, the patient and your physician should make the ultimate decision for the use of the drug. Together you should evaluate the risk factor and likelihood of its benefit.

❤   ❤   ❤

Everyone only goes around the track once in life,
and if you don't enjoy that trip, it's pretty pathetic.
- Gary Rogers -

🖤 🖤 🖤

Subject: Paradox
Author: Unknown
"The Paradox", dedicated by a radio station in Nashville, TN to the memory of those who lost their lives at Columbine High School, Littleton, Colorado, on April 20, 1999, and to the family and friends who are left behind...

The Paradox

THE PARADOX OF OUR TIME IN HISTORY IS THAT WE HAVE TALLER BUILDINGS, BUT SHORTER TEMPERS; WIDER FREEWAYS, BUT NARROWER VIEWPOINTS; WE SPEND MORE, BUT HAVE LESS; WE BUY MORE, BUT ENJOY IT LESS.

WE HAVE BIGGER HOUSES AND SMALLER FAMILIES; MORE CONVENIENCES, BUT LESS TIME; WE HAVE MORE DEGREES, BUT LESS SENSE; MORE KNOWLEDGE, BUT LESS JUDGMENT; MORE EXPERTS, BUT MORE PROBLEMS; MORE MEDICINE, BUT LESS WELLNESS.

WE HAVE MULTIPLIED OUR POSSESSIONS, BUT REDUCED OUR VALUES. WE TALK TOO MUCH, LOVE TOO SELDOM, AND HATE TOO OFTEN. WE LEARNED HOW TO MAKE A LIVING, BUT NOT A LIFE. WE'VE ADDED YEARS TO LIFE, NOT LIFE TO YEARS.

WE'VE BEEN ALL THE WAY TO THE MOON AND BACK, BUT HAVE TROUBLE CROSSING THE STREET TO MEET THE NEW NEIGHBOR. WE'VE CONQUERED OUTER SPACE, BUT NOT INNER SPACE; WE'VE CLEANED UP THE AIR, BUT POL-LUTED THE SOUL; WE'VE SPLIT THE ATOM, BUT NOT OUR PREJUDICE; WE HAVE HIGHER INCOMES, BUT LOWER MOR-ALS; WE'VE BECOME LONG ON QUANTITY, BUT SHORT ON QUALITY.

THESE ARE THE TIMES OF TALL MEN, AND SHORT CHAR-ACTER; STEEP PROFITS, AND SHALLOW RELATIONSHIPS.

THESE ARE THE TIMES OF WORLD PEACE, BUT DOMESTIC WARFARE; MORE LEISURE, BUT LESS FUN; MORE KINDS OF FOOD, BUT LESS NUTRITION.

THESE ARE THE DAYS OF TWO INCOMES, BUT MORE DIVORCE; OF FANCIER HOUSES, BUT BROKEN HOMES.

IT IS A TIME WHEN THERE IS MUCH IN THE SHOW WINDOW AND NOTHING IN THE STOCKROOM;

A TIME WHEN TECHNOLOGY CAN BRING THIS LETTER TO YOU, AND A TIME WHEN YOU CAN CHOOSE EITHER TO MAKE A DIFFERENCE OR JUST HIT DELETE.

❤ ❤ ❤

Heal the past, live the present, dream the future.
(Credited to Mary Engelbreit)

CHAPTER 43

Taking responsibility for your own actions

In a meeting the other day, a coworker said to me "I need to have you do something for me." I innocently responded, "What would that be?" It turned out this person was falling behind on a project that she committed to, but had now realized she did not have time to complete it on schedule. Her annual bonus was tied directly into her finishing this very important (to her) project...and if she didn't complete it, she would not receive the substantial monetary reward. Having my own projects to complete, I calmly stated I would not be able to assist her. She then turned to the other members of the group and proceeded to COMMAND them to assist her, which they all declined to do. Gracefully I may add, but decline they did. It was obvious from the beginning that she wore her intentions on her blouse sleeves. She had developed a poor reputation for only thinking about her own priorities and was known for not being a team player. From my experience, people tend not to want to help those that don't want to help themselves.

Have you ever been around selfish folks that only have their own agenda in mind, and could care less about you or me? Sure. It happens all the time.

What if someone had taken her up on her "demand" to bail her out of her problem? What untold stress would that have placed on everyone concerned? None for her, but for the rest who bought into her childish tactics, tons.

Could she have handled this dilemma more effectively, with more compassion, and ultimately with a better outcome? You bet. Being put into this situation, and I was pressed with a deadline to complete a project, I would have "asked" for assistance...with full disclosure WHY I needed help. Perhaps, if the bonus were large enough, I would have said I would be happy to share the bonus with all the members of the team. Volunteering to take some project in the future would be in order. "You help me now with an IOU for later" type of arrangement would be more appropriate.

We all get in tight spots where we need assistance from time to time, but we should always take full and complete responsibility for our actions, no matter the consequences.

There is a direct correlation between the level of responsibility for one's illness and the rate at which you recover. I knew a co-worker at the company I used to work for that fell short of his responsibility to his family...by committing suicide. By him not seeing any other way out but the path he took, he deprived his family and friends of his love and companionship for years to come. He failed to take responsibility for whatever ailed him (or trouble he had gotten himself into), and left the task of raising his children to those around him.

We have a friend that has just found out she has MS (Multiple Sclerosis). She and her husband have taken absolute responsibility for every aspect of her "wellness" campaign. They are both attacking this illness as one would do in a military campaign, and will do anything to conquer this disease. The operative words here are "ABSOLUTE RESPONSIBILITY". The interesting thing about this couple, over that of the first example, is that by them helping themselves, other people have rallied around them to assist. When I had my heart attack, I didn't expect others to take responsibility for my recovery. Sure, I expected the doctors to do what they were trained to do...which was to bring me back from death's door. But I took control of the situation after that, being responsible for my own recovery was my problem, and no one else's. Did I have the help, love, concern and devotion from my family? Yes. But if I had not stepped up to the bar and put myself in the driver's seat, I am convinced that no one else would have been so open to assist.

So what are the benefits of taking control of my health care decisions? Once I made the decision to become fully recovered, I experienced less anxiety. My mental attitude improved...helping to increase my own body's healing properties. Because I was completely committed and actively involved and participating in returning to a normal life, my whole body joined in on the fight to recovery. My doctor told me what to expect in the days, weeks, and months ahead, what my limitations would be, and what I could expect to realistically see as the end result of my mental and physical recovery plan. I recovered fully because I had solid and obtainable goals to shoot for.

By becoming more self-sufficient, you must take complete ownership of your actions, and their consequences. You need to develop your ability to perceive yourself as the "driver" of your own fate, and the controller of your own destiny. The ultimate benefits for creating more responsibility, and hence, relying less on the resources of others, will enhance your existence, build self worth, which in turn will provide your life with fulfillment and meaning.

♥   ♥   ♥

IF I HAD MY LIFE TO LIVE OVER
by Erma Bombeck

(Written after she found out she was dying from cancer.)

I WOULD HAVE GONE TO BED WHEN I WAS SICK INSTEAD OF PRETENDING THE EARTH WOULD GO INTO A HOLDING PATTERN IF I WEREN'T THERE FOR THE DAY.

I WOULD HAVE BURNED THE PINK CANDLE SCULPTED LIKE A ROSE BEFORE IT MELTED IN STORAGE.

I WOULD HAVE TALKED LESS AND LISTENED MORE. I WOULD HAVE INVITED FRIENDS OVER TO DINNER EVEN IF THE CARPET WAS STAINED, OR THE SOFA FADED.

I WOULD HAVE EATEN THE POPCORN IN THE 'GOOD' LIVING ROOM AND WORRIED MUCH LESS ABOUT THE DIRT WHEN SOMEONE WANTED TO LIGHT A FIRE IN THE FIREPLACE.

I WOULD HAVE TAKEN THE TIME TO LISTEN TO MY GRANDFATHER RAMBLE ABOUT HIS YOUTH.

I WOULD NEVER HAVE INSISTED THE CAR WINDOWS BE ROLLED UP ON A SUMMER DAY BECAUSE MY HAIR HAD JUST BEEN TEASED AND SPRAYED.

I WOULD HAVE SAT ON THE LAWN WITH MY CHILDREN AND NOT WORRIED ABOUT GRASS STAINS.

I WOULD HAVE CRIED AND LAUGHED LESS WHILE WATCHING TELEVISION-AND MORE WHILE WATCHING LIFE.

I WOULD NEVER HAVE BOUGHT ANYTHING JUST BECAUSE IT WAS PRACTICAL, WOULDN'T SHOW SOIL, OR WAS GUARANTEED TO LAST A LIFETIME.

INSTEAD OF WISHING AWAY NINE MONTHS OF PREGNANCY, I'D HAVE CHERISHED EVERY MOMENT AND REALIZED THAT THE WONDERMENT GROWING INSIDE ME WAS THE ONLY CHANCE IN LIFE TO ASSIST GOD IN A MIRACLE.

WHEN MY KIDS KISSED ME IMPETUOUSLY, I WOULD NEVER HAVE SAID, "LATER. NOW GO GET WASHED UP FOR DINNER."

THERE WOULD HAVE BEEN MORE "I LOVE YOU'S." MORE "I'M SORRY'S."

BUT MOSTLY, GIVEN ANOTHER SHOT AT LIFE, I WOULD SEIZE EVERY MINUTE...LOOK AT IT AND REALLY SEE IT ... LIVE IT...AND NEVER GIVE IT BACK.

STOP SWEATING THE SMALL STUFF. DON'T WORRY ABOUT WHO DOESN'T LIKE YOU, WHO HAS MORE, OR WHO'S DOING WHAT.

INSTEAD, LET'S CHERISH THE RELATIONSHIPS WE HAVE WITH THOSE WHO DO LOVE US. LET'S THINK ABOUT WHAT GOD HAS BLESSED US WITH.

AND WHAT WE ARE DOING EACH DAY TO PROMOTE OURSELVES MENTALLY, PHYSICALLY, EMOTIONALLY, AS WELL AS SPIRITUALLY.

LIFE IS TOO SHORT TO LET IT PASS YOU BY. WE ONLY HAVE ONE SHOT AT THIS AND THEN IT'S GONE. I HOPE YOU ALL HAVE A BLESSED DAY.

(IN MEMORY OF ERMA BOMBECK WHO LOST HER FIGHT WITH CANCER.)

CHAPTER 44

One last thing - before I go

This is your life. No one else shares your thoughts, dreams, concerns, loves, cares, family and friends as much as you do. As you know by now, my wife Beth will probably never have a heart attack like I did. She is a living-breathing example of every lesson given in this dissertation. She loves, and is loved, cares about people (friends, acquaintances, and strangers) with the same degree of intensity. She never gets mad at people on the freeway that cut her off (unlike what I used to do), never keeps things bottled up inside her until she "bursts", and she flows with the multitude of changes that come her way with ease.

Over the years, I have watched, learned, and mostly emulated her, and discovered with amazement that for the most part, she, as well as women worldwide, know more than they are letting on. Just watch a mom dealing with the rigors of her "life" for 24 hours, and you will develop a major appreciation for how multi-tasking they really are.

After watching my wife, and my two grown daughters, Kelly and Kimberly with their own kids, I started to understand how truly talented they, as well as most women are at the day-to-day running of their lives. With the baby in one arm, phone cradled in the nap of the neck, talking to someone on the phone...while at the same time standing at the stove cooking breakfast for the young ones...neither of them have ever stressed out, or lost their cool or composure.

Don't get me wrong; we men are amazing at what we do. We are achievers, builders of empires, and creators of all things magnificent. But so are the women of the world. They do things that we could never do...no matter how hard we work. They create life, nurture that life, care for and love that life, until that new life can stand on his/her own two feet.

But here is the difference between them and us. We (men) have more heart disease than they do. Why? I venture to guess that women see the same problem totally differently then men do. As Dr. John Grey states from the book of the same name, *"Men are from Mars and Women are from Venus"*. Perhaps the approaches that women take to solve problems ARE different from the way we men solve problems. I know for a fact that my wife looks at problems totally differently from the way I do, and handles it accordingly, without stress, or anger. She just does what it takes to deal with it, resolves it quickly, and moves on.

The point I am trying to make is this. From my experience, we men have an ego that, at times, may get us in trouble. I saw the heart attack coming, and did nothing about it. Only after I keeled over in the back seat of our car, did I finally realize that something may be happening to me that was out of the ordinary. We were lucky the first time around. We may not be so lucky again...if we don't change...and change fast.

I have outlined - through essays, anecdotes, humor, and a few facts, the seriousness of what you and I have been through. Life can be hard, at times...and wonderful, too. Life can be a feast to be savored, or a desolate wind-blown desert, full of land mines, no water, or shade to keep you cool.

Or it can be an Oasis. It's your choice.

You may find that by testing out some of my theories, you see a change in the way you accomplish your tasks. By swimming with the current, but controlling the flow of the river, you get something done, but with less stress, and you accomplish it more quickly and get farther along than you ever dreamed possible. By dealing with unresolved issues of anger, you become more peaceful, your blood pressure stays low, you don't swear as much, and loved ones respond to you differently than they normally have in the past.

You may find that by changing your attitude, you change your heart. You see your neighbors differently, and your relationship with your loved ones becomes stronger, more loving and your level of stress at the office diminish - all because you have taken back control of your own destiny.

Because you now look at fear differently than you did before you picked up *Heart Attack Survivor - a field guide*, you see that fear for what it really is - something to go through, and not be stopped by. Remember, you are not alone. Me, you, and a lot of other wonderful folks survived heart disease.

Thanks to our family and our friends, we are now on the road to recovery. Better than we were before!!

One last thing - before I go. This life you now fully own should never be squandered. It's a gift to be cherished, savored, and held on to. You have the absolute right to enjoy it to the fullest. I hope this book has been useful and will be for years to come.

At the end of our days, it's not the things we do that we regret.
It's the things we didn't do.
- Beth Henson-

EASY ORDER FORM

Make checks or Money orders payable to the author:

BRAD HENSON and send to

Crow Publishing
2510-G Las Posas Rd. #260
Camarillo, California

Or Fax to 415-329-3291

QTY		Price each	Total
	Heart Attack Survivor	$19.95	
	Sales Tax (CA residents 7.25%)		
	Shipping/Handling ($3 for first item; add $1.75 for each additional item)		
	Total		

Name: _____

Address: _____

City: _____ State _____ Zip: _____

Phone: (   ): _____

Fax: (   ): _____

E-Mail Address: _____

Credit Card Number: _____

Exp. Date_____

Name (as it appears on card): _____

You may also order the book " Heart Attack Survivor a field guide" by going to our website at the following URL:
www.heartattacksurvivor.com
to place the order for faster turn-a-round or order from other online book sellers of your choice.

EASY ORDER FORM

Make checks or Money orders payable to the author:

BRAD HENSON and send to

Crow Publishing
2510-G Las Posas Rd. #260
Camarillo, California

Or Fax to 415-329-3291

QTY		Price each	Total
	Heart Attack Survivor	$19.95	
	Sales Tax (CA residents 7.25%)		
	Shipping/Handling ($3 for first item; add $1.75 for each additional item)		
	Total		

Name: _____

Address: _____

City: _____ State _____ Zip: _____

Phone: ( ): _____

Fax: ( ): _____

E-Mail Address: _____

Credit Card Number: _____

Exp. Date_____

Name (as it appears on card): _____

You may also order the book " Heart Attack Survivor a field guide" by going to our website at the following URL:

www.heartattacksurvivor.com

to place the order for faster turn-a-round or order from other online book sellers of your choice.

NOTES

Printed in the United States
20392LVS00002B/331

9 780971 278806